EMERGENCY TELEPHONE NUMBERS

Doctor: _____

Poison Control Center: _____

Ambulance: _____

Taxi: _____

Hospital: _____

Neighbor: _____

Mother: _____   work: _____

Father: _____   work: _____

A PARENTS' GUIDE TO POISNS IN THE HOME

*The Essential Sourcebook
on Toxic Household Products*

GIDEON KOREN, MD

GRAMERCY BOOKS
NEW YORK • AVENEL

Published by Gramercy Books,
Random House Value Publishing, Inc.
40 Engelhard Avenue,
Avenel, New Jersey 07001.

Random House
New York • Toronto • London • Sydney • Auckland

Printed and bound in the United States

Library of Congress Cataloging–in–Publication Data
Koren, Gideon,   1947–
The parents' guide to poisons in the home : the essential
sourcebook on toxic household products / Gideon Koren.
                    p.   cm.
                 Includes index.
            ISBN 0–517–14812–9
      1. Toxicology—Popular works.   I. Title.
         RE1213.K67   1995
         615.9—dc20   95–22144
                                    CIP
The material contained in this book is intended as a
guideline only. The publisher and
author assume no responsibility for death or injuries
incurred using the information herein. Please consult your
physician, hospital emergency department, or poison
control center.

Stoddart Publishing gratefully acknowledges the support
of the Canada Council, Ontario Ministry of Culture,
Tourism, and Recreation, Ontario Arts Council, and
Ontario Publishing Centre in the development of writing
and publishing in Canada.

Published by arrangement with the Stoddart Publishing Co.

First Gramercy Books reprint edition: © 1995

8 7 6 5 4 3 2 1

CONTENTS

INTRODUCTION

As a parent or caregiver, you want to keep your children safe from harm and do all you can to ensure they grow up to become healthy, happy adults. As a pediatrician, toxicologist, and father of four, I share this goal with you, and know well the fears and guilt parents experience after a child has ingested a toxic substance. I've written *The Parents' Guide to Poisons in the Home* because I want to spare children and parents the tragedies my colleagues and I have witnessed during the years at our hospital. This book includes not only preventive measures, but up-to-date advice on first aid for poisoning, with a focus on the actions parents or caregivers can take.

Every year more than half a million children under the age of six are reported to poison control centers in North America after exposure to toxic substances both inside and outside the home. Of these, several hundred die or are left with permanent damage — which in many cases could have been prevented, had the necessary steps been taken. An accidental poisoning can occur despite the most vigilant of parents and the most protected of environments, for even seemingly harmless substances can be poisonous in large quantities.

Of the children experiencing serious poisoning, one-third are between one and two years old; almost two-thirds are between one and three — the so-called terrible twos. With their newly acquired motor independence but not yet the common sense and insight that are achieved and developed during the preschool years (age four to six), these young children want to try everything, for that is how they learn about the world, and the contents of cabinets, drawers, and purses hold great allure.

Read Pages 1 to 8 of this book now, rather than waiting until there's a crisis. The instructions therein may save the life of your child in the future.

Gideon Koren, M.D.

HOW TO USE THIS BOOK

While *The Parents' Guide to Poisons in the Home* cannot and should not replace consultation with your doctor or with a poison control center, it is designed to familiarize you with the simple steps you can take to prevent an accidental poisoning or, if one occurs, what effective immediate actions you can take. In a time of crisis it is difficult to cope with complex, lengthy explanations. Therefore, I have kept information to the bare essentials, and organized it into three parts.

The first section focuses on *what you should know now* in terms of preventing and managing poisoning. When it comes to accidental poisoning, the only sure cure is prevention. I have outlined the practical steps you can take to prevent poisoning in the first place. In addition, I have described some first-aid techniques, including cardiopulmonary resuscitation.

The next section is an alphabetical listing, including description and procedures, of the most common poisons children ingest or encounter. Both prescription and over-the-counter drugs, household chemicals, cosmetics, plants, and snake and spider venom are covered. The list of drugs and chemicals is by no means comprehensive, for there are thousands in this category and room for only some of them in this book. To decide which to include, I chose substances that:
— have been reported to cause severe poisoning or death in children;
— have been commonly ingested by children; and
— can kill even in small doses.

Some common trade names are given, as well as information on what the substance is used for, the signs of poisoning, what to do if your child ingests it — depending on whether you are close to or far from medical help — what dosage is toxic, and the effect of the substance. The toxicity of each substance is indicated by asterisks:

*   **Safe or very rarely causes major effects on health**
**   **Can have major effects on health, but rarely causes death**
***   **Has major effects on health and death is not uncommon**
**** **Commonly results in death.**

Starting on page 113 is a comprehensive listing of poison control centers with phone numbers.

Finally, you will find an index with a full alphabetical listing of brand names and generic names of chemicals, plants, animals, and drugs. If you know the name of the chemical or drug your child has ingested, you can look it up here. Page references will lead you to the section that deals with the substance.

AN OUNCE OF PREVENTION:
WHAT YOU NEED TO DO NOW

The following information may save the life of your child. Read these pages as if your child's life depended on it, and then follow the instructions. Remember, the only sure cure for poisoning is prevention.

SAFEGUARDING YOUR CHILD AGAINST POISONS

1. Poison-Proof Your Home
The most important thing to keep in mind when poison-proofing your home is that *if children can reach the substance, they may swallow it.* With this in mind:

- Place all drugs and chemicals well out of the reach of your child, in *locked* cabinets, suitcases, or boxes.
- Store all drugs and chemicals in child-proof containers and *never* in old pop bottles or jars normally used for food.
- Clearly label contents and mark containers POISON, even substances that seem innocent, such as your iron pills. Iron pills cause more than 2000 poisonings in young children every year, and about a dozen die every year from major complications.
- Take drugs that have expired or chemicals no longer used to your local toxic-waste centre. Never pour them down drains, toilets, or throw them in the garbage.
- Return drugs and chemicals to safe storage immediately after use. Substances left "for only a minute" can kill in seconds.
- Be especially careful if you live with or visit elderly people. The elderly tend to take more medications, which are often stored in containers that are not child-proof.
- Don't leave medications on night tables or in your purse.
- Always turn on the light when taking or giving medications at night.
- Read labels twice to make sure you are giving a sick child the right medication or dose.
- Never call medicine "candy."
- Don't allow children to play with medication or chemical containers.

- Make sure any household your child may visit, or the day-care center, is safe.
- Don't keep poisonous plants in your home.

These rules may seem self-evident. Yet many of us don't follow them. Take your kitchen, for example. Toddlers love to open cupboards and play with pots and bowls. How many of us keep cleaning supplies such as bleach, drain cleaners, and lye, which can cause terrible damage, just beneath the sink? And how many of us store dangerous chemicals such as insecticides in our garage?

2. Poison-Proof Your Garden and Garage

- Know which insects, spiders, or snakes in your area may be poisonous.
- Learn what plants, if any, in your garden are poisonous, then either remove them or keep a vigilant eye on small children playing in the garden.
- In your garage store chemicals in locked cabinets, suitcases, or boxes, including high cupboards that may seem out of reach. Children have astonishing climbing abilities!

WHAT TO DO IN CASE OF POISONING

Parents need to become familiar with the steps to take if a child ingests poison. This is the aim of this section, but the best thing you can do for yourself and your family is to take courses in first aid and CPR (cardiopulmonary resuscitation). Not only will you know what to do if needed, you will be less likely to panic and therefore more capable of determining the severity of a situation.

THE ABCs OF LIFE SUPPORT

Life support should always come first. The ABCs of life support are:

Airway. Check to see if the child's airway is open and free. Open the mouth and remove any substances. Use a light source (e.g., flashlight) if you have one. Remove the substance (a tablet, a plant leaf) as carefully as possible. The child may struggle and may not let you open his mouth. Don't give up until you are sure that anything you can remove is out.

Breathing. Is the child breathing? Watch the movement of the chest. As you can see in Table 1, the normal respiratory rate (number of breaths per minute) varies with age.

Table 1: Changes in respiratory rate according to age

Age	Respiratory rate (breaths per minute)
At birth	30
5 yrs	24
10 yrs	20
15 yrs	16
Adults	12

If the child is not breathing, you must start *artificial respiration* (see Figure 1) immediately, because the body cannot survive more than a few minutes without oxygen. Mouth-to-mouth resuscitation is the best method. Blow air into the child's mouth (while blocking the nose, so air will not come out) or into the child's nose (while blocking the mouth). Watch the child's chest to ensure it expands, and then release the nostrils or mouth and allow the air to come out. Count 1 while blowing in and then 2, 3, 4, 5 while you allow the air to come out — about 4 seconds per cycle.

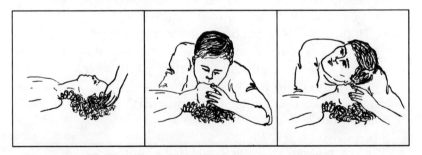

Figure 1. (a) Open child's mouth and remove any foreign objects. Then tilt head back. (b) Pinch child's nostrils shut between your thumb and index finger. Take a breath and place your mouth over the child's mouth. Blow air into the child's mouth. Observe if chest rises. (c) Remove your mouth and fingers. Listen for air being exhaled. Repeat until child begins to breathe on her own.

Cardiovascular. Is the child's heart beating? The simplest way to tell is by feeling the pulse at the wrist. Lack of pulse does not necessarily mean that the heart is not beating; it may still be pumping blood, but at a very low pressure, which occurs when someone goes into shock. Check for a more central pulse, such as the neck arteries.

If there is no heartbeat, start external cardiac massage. Figure 2 shows you how this is done.

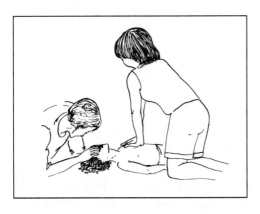

Figure 2. External cardiac massage is done when the child has no heartbeat. Place the child on a hard surface. Sitting on your knees on the right side of the child, place your hands on his sternum (middle chest bone), with the heel of one hand just over the lower border of the sternum and the other hand on top of the first. Compress the heart by pressing your hands against the sternum in short strokes a half second long. Repeat 80 times a minute.

If the child is not breathing, too (which is often the case), one person should do mouth-to-mouth respiration (see Figure 1) while another does the cardiac massage.

If the child is not breathing and has no pulse, cardiac massage must be performed simultaneously with mouth-to-mouth respiration as shown in Figure 2.

If the child is or becomes unconscious at home, rush her to the closest medical facility. If you are alone with the child, call a neighbour to drive while you constantly ensure the child is breathing and has a pulse. If she does not, you need to initiate CPR immediately. Every second is important.

Table 2: First Aid as Related to Poisoning

---

1) Check the ABCs: *Airway, Breathing, and Cardiovascular.*
2) Try to identify *what* the child was exposed to.
3) Try to determine *how much* the child consumed.

4) Remove unswallowed substance from mouth or wash from skin.
5) Call physician or poison control center.
6) Look up substance in this book to see what can be done immediately while waiting for professional assistance.

IDENTIFY THE POISON
Try to determine what the child drank or chewed, or what has spilled onto his skin or in his eyes. This is very important because different poisons require different treatments. For example, if the child swallowed kerosene or gasoline, you should not make him vomit, because the vapors could damage the lungs. *Always* take the container with you to the hospital or to the medical facility.

ESTIMATE THE AMOUNT OF POISON INGESTED
Generally, the more poison the child swallows or inhales, the greater the damage. Therefore, you should try to determine how much of the toxic substance the child was exposed to. For example, if a bottle of 40 iron pills bought only yesterday now has only 20 pills, then you will have to assume that the child consumed 20 pills, unless you find some of them on the floor. Sometimes you may not be sure how many tablets or how much liquid the child has swallowed. Just do your best.

DECONTAMINATE
Decontamination means cleaning or minimizing the exposure of the child to the poison. You can do this by, for example:
— *removing* tablets or parts of pills from the mouth or a poisonous spider from the child's arm.
— washing the skin, mouth, or eyes with lots of water at room temperature if the child spills a chemical on himself. Washing not only removes the material, but also dilutes the poison.
— inducing vomiting. After a child has swallowed a substance, you need to act quickly to minimize the absorption of chemicals into the body. But check this book or call your poison control centre first, because in some cases vomiting may do more harm than good.
The best way to induce vomiting is with syrup of ipecac (pronounced i-pi-kak). This compound, prepared from a plant, will

induce vomiting in almost everyone if given in the right dose. Keep a 30-mL bottle of ipecac locked in your medicine cabinet.

Table 3: Amount of Ipecac Needed to Induce Vomiting

Age	Amount
under 1	5 mL (1 tsp)
1-4	10 mL (2 tsp)
4-12	15 mL (3 tsp)
teenager/adult	15-30 mL (1-2 tbsp)

Ipecac should be followed by a small amount of pop, milk, or water. Vomiting will generally occur within 10-20 minutes. If not, repeat the dose.

If you do not have syrup of ipecac at home, liquid detergent has been shown in recent studies to work well. Use 5-15 mL (1-3 tsp).

If you are not at home and none of the above is at hand, or if the child refuses to swallow, insert a finger into the child's throat. This simple means can cause vomiting.

Do *not* induce vomiting if the child

— is not fully conscious. The vomited material may be aspirated, or breathed, into the lungs, a very dangerous situation.
— is convulsing, because vomiting worsens the convulsion.
— has ingested corrosives (alkali or acid) because they will cause further damage to the esophagus, throat, and mouth.
— has ingested petroleum products (lighter fluid, paint thinners or removers, kerosene, gasoline, etc.), because during vomiting their vapors (fumes) will be inhaled and cause damage to the respiratory system.

WHAT HAPPENS AT THE HOSPITAL

Once your child arrives at the hospital, health professionals will take over.

During the first few hours after ingesting poison, a trained medical team will attempt to remove as much of the ingested material as possible. They do this by nasogastric lavage, commonly called stomach pumping, which is a method of inserting a tube through the nose and down the esophagus to the stomach, and then sucking out the contents. Clean water is poured in and sucked out again, until only clear water comes out. A trained medical team is needed to ensure minimal trauma to the child.

Certain materials can prevent the absorption of chemicals from the gut. The most widely used is *activated charcoal,* which has tremendous capacity to bind many different drugs or chemicals and prevent their absorption into the body. Activated charcoal, generally combined with a cathartic (which hastens exit from the body by causing diarrhea), is a safe material that comes in 25–40-g containers and can be bought in pharmacies. Each 10 g of charcoal should be mixed with 100 mL (⅓ cup) of tap water. So if the bottle has, for example, 40 g charcoal, then 400 mL (1 ¾ cups) of water are needed. The solution must be mixed thoroughly. The most difficult part is getting the child to drink the solution. In most cases it has to be given in the emergency room through a nasogastric tube. But if the child is co-operative, you may try to get him to sip the solution. Do not try more than 300 mL (up to about one glassful).

Different doctors have different views about whether or not parents should administer charcoal. For example, if you live far away from a medical facility, it may be more important to give charcoal yourself than if you live in the city. If you have more experience — for instance, if you are a child-care worker or health professional — the procedure may be easier.

Consult your physician, pharmacist, and poison control center about this possibility.

After pumping the stomach and giving an activated-charcoal solution, the doctor concentrates on minimizing the effects of absorbed poisons by using *antidotes.* Antidotes are chemicals that neutralize the effect of a specific poison, either in the gut before it is absorbed, or when it is in the body. Most antidotes are strong medications that have their own side effects and therefore must be administered by an experienced medical team.

In some cases the doctor tries to minimize the damage by increasing the excretion of poisons through the kidneys, both by increasing urine output and by changing its acidity (pH). If the kidneys are not functioning because of the poisoning or complications, then dialysis may have to be used.

Other poisons may need to be removed by *hemoperfusion.* In this procedure the blood of the patient is passed through materials such as charcoal that can bind the poison, thus removing it from the blood.

Often there are no specific antidotes for a given drug or chemical. In such cases, the medical team simply maintains body functions until the poison has left the system or until the damage is repaired. For example, if a child has inhaled gasoline fumes, she may be kept on oxygen or given chest physiotherapy to minimize damage to the lungs.

EMERGENCY TREATMENT FOR COMMON POISONS

This section contains an alphabetical listing of the generic, or scientific, names of common toxic substances. If you know only the brand, or commercial, name of a drug (for example, Tylenol), you need to check the index for the page reference. Note that many of the commercial names include all or part of the generic name.

Unfortunately this list cannot include all the drugs on the market. If the name does not appear, read the label for the active ingredient and find it in the index.

Also included are poisonous plants that children commonly ingest and information on what to do if your child is bitten by a spider, scorpion, or snake. Only the signs of poisoning likely to be helpful to the adult who has no medical background are described. For other signs and symptoms you may consult other texts and the information sheet that generally comes with a drug when you purchase it. Remember, when a child is poisoned, *not all the signs described for a specific poisoning may appear. Sometimes no signs at all appear, and sometimes only one or two.*

Table 4: Non-Poisonous Products Children Often Ingest[*]

The following chemicals are not poisonous (that is, have not been shown to cause permanent or serious health effects) *unless swallowed or ingested in very large amounts.* Nevertheless, the child may feel ill, and you should seek medical attention without delay.

Adhesives (glues)
Antacids
Bath oil (castor oil and perfume)
Body lotion
Calamine lotion
Candles
Chalk
Cigarettes and cigars
Clay
Cologne
Contraceptive pills
Crayons

Deodorants
Deodorizers (room and refrigerator)
Grease
Hand lotion and creams
Hydrogen peroxide (3%)
Ink
Laxatives
Lipstick
Lubricants
Make-up
Matches
Mineral oil
Pencils
Perfume
Play-Doh
Rouge
Rubber cement
Sachets
Shampoo
Shaving cream and lotion
Soap
Suntan/sunblock preparations
Sweetening agents (Saccharin, Sugartwin, Equal, etc.)
Toothpaste
Vaseline
Watercolour paints

---

* Adapted from Mofenson et al, Emerg Med North America 1984; 2:162, WB Saunders, Philadelphia.

***ACETAMINOPHEN

COMMERCIAL NAMES
Acetaco, Algisin, Amacodone, Amaphen, Anacin (also name used for aspirin, check active ingredient), Anoquan, Bancap, Banex, Codalin, Co-Gastric, Compal, Comtrex, Cals Cogeopinin, Damcet, Darvocet, Dolecet, Dorcol, Dristan, Empracet, Espig, Excedrin, G1, G-2, G-3, Hydrocet, Larcet, Lortab, Medilgeric, Midol, Migralam, Pacaps, Panadol, Parafon, Paralgin, Percocet, Phrenilin, Propocet, Protid, Sedapan, Tralgon, Tylenol, Valadol.

USE
Acetaminophen is the most widely used drug for fever and pain in children. It is also widely used by adults.

LEVEL OF DANGER
Life may be in danger if amounts greater than 100 mg per kg (2 lb) of body weight, or 3 regular adult Tylenol tablets/caplets, or 11 pediatric Tylenols taken by a toddler weighing 10 kg (22 lb) or less.

SIGNS OF POISONING (not all signs have to be present)
Pallor; nausea; vomiting; drowsiness, and mental confusion. If there has been damage to the liver, the signs take a day or more to show. These may include pain and tenderness of right upper abdomen, yellow tinge to skin (jaundice), drowsiness, and loss of consciousness.

WHAT TO DO FOR PREVENTION
If your child is being treated with acetaminophen for illness, be sure to discuss with your physician or pharmacist the exact dose the child needs, the interactions that may occur with other drugs, and side effects of chronic use. Be extremely careful to give the correct dose when switching from liquid to tablets, or vice versa.

WHAT DO TO IN CASE OF POISONING
1. Remove remaining tablets from the child's mouth.
2. Ensure that the child is breathing and has a heartbeat (see page 3).
3. Induce vomiting with ipecac (see page 5). If the child is sleepy,

unconscious, already vomiting, or has had a seizure, do not give ipecac.
4. Take the child to hospital as soon as possible.
5. Bring with you the drug container and try to estimate how much acetaminophen the child has swallowed.

****ACIDS

USE
Acids are used as metal cleaners, soldering fluxes, automobile battery fluid, swimming-pool sanitizers, bleaches. Children commonly ingest drain cleaners, toilet bowl cleaners, anti-rust compounds or industrial cleaners, which contain strong acids.

LEVEL OF DANGER
Even small amounts can cause major damage or be life-threatening to small children.

SIGNS OF POISONING (not all signs have to be present)
Severe pain in mouth, throat, chest, and/or stomach; drooling; nausea and vomiting; diarrhea with very dark stool (indicates presence of blood); irritation and peeling of the lining of the mouth and throat; difficulty in breathing; twitching; seizures; weak pulse; and loss of consciousness.

WHAT TO DO IN CASE OF POISONING
1. Ensure that the child is breathing and has a heartbeat (see page 3).
2. *Do not* try to induce vomiting, because this will cause further damage to the alimentary tract.
3. Give the child milk or water to drink to neutralize and dilute the acid.
4. Wash the acid carefully with a large amount of water from all areas it may have contacted (e.g., face, arms, and eyes).
5. If the child has difficulty breathing (due to swelling of throat), rush her to the nearest medical facility.
6. If the child is in pain, give acetaminophen (e.g., Tylenol) or acetaminophen with codeine.
7. Take the child to the nearest medical facility.
8. Bring with you the substance container, and try to estimate how much the child has swallowed.

*ADHESIVES (Glues)

LEVEL OF DANGER
Adhesives contain various organic solvents, such as toluene, benzene, xylene, acetone, and hexane. The amount of glue a child may ingest is rarely enough to be life-threatening. The dangerous dose is generally 0.2 g per kg (2.2 lb) of body weight.

SIGNS OF POISONING (not all signs have to be present)
Mouth and throat irritation, dizziness, weakness, euphoria, nausea and vomiting, headache, unsteadiness, tremors, slow and shallow breathing, changes in heart rate, excited or violent behaviour, loss of consciousness.

WHAT TO DO IN CASE OF POISONING
1. *Do not* try to induce vomiting, because of risk of further damage to alimentary tract or of inhaling solvents.
2. Give the child milk or water to drink.
3. Take the child to hospital as soon as possible.
4. Bring with you the adhesive substance container and try to estimate the amount the child has swallowed.

***AKEE

BACKGROUND
This is a tropical plant (*Blighia sophida*) that grows in the Caribbean and southern Florida. The fruit is eaten mainly in Jamaica. Its unripened fruit and cotyledons (first leaves) are poisonous.

LEVEL OF DANGER
One unripe fruit can kill a child. In Jamaica there are several deaths every year, especially in children.

SIGNS OF POISONING (not all signs have to be present)
Nausea, vomiting, and abdominal pain within two hours; after an "improvement," there is a second, more violent attack, with seizures, loss of consciousness, hypoglycaemia, and deep coma.

WHAT TO DO FOR PREVENTION
1. Do not allow children to touch unripened fruit.
2. Immediately discard water used to cook the fruits.

WHAT TO DO IN CASE OF POISONING
1. Remove remaining substance from mouth.
2. Ensure that the child is breathing and has a heartbeat (see page 3).
3. Induce vomiting with ipecac (see page 5). If the child is sleepy or unconscious, already vomiting, or has had a seizure, do not give ipecac.
4. Take the child to hospital as soon as possible.
5. Bring with you remnants of the fruit and try to estimate how much the child has swallowed.

****ALKALIS

USE
Alkalis are used in the manufacture of soaps and cleaners. They are found in batteries, drain cleaners, household ammonia, automatic-dishwasher detergents, oven cleaners, bleaches, metal cleaners containing ammonia, paint removers, and washing powders.

LEVEL OF DANGER
Ingestion of alkalis can be life-threatening, and even a small amount can cause permanent damage. The child may suffer narrowing of the esophagus because of scarring.

SIGNS OF POISONING (not all signs have to be present)
Severe pain in the mouth, throat, chest, and/or stomach; drooling; visible irritation and peeling of the lining of the mouth and throat; difficulty in breathing; nausea and vomiting; diarrhea with very dark stool (indicates presence of blood); rapid and weak pulse; and loss of consciousness.

WHAT TO DO IN CASE OF POISONING
1. Ensure that the child is breathing and has a pulse (see page 3).
2. *Do not* try to induce vomiting, because this will cause further damage to the alimentary tract.
3. Give the child milk or water to drink to neutralize and dilute the alkali.
4. Wash the alkali carefully with large amounts of water from all areas it may have contacted (e.g., face, arms, and eyes).
5. If the child has difficulty breathing (due to swelling of throat), rush him to the nearest medical facility.
6. If the child is in pain, give him acetaminophen (e.g., Tylenol) or acetaminophen with codeine.
7. Take the child to hospital as quickly as possible.
8. Bring with you the substance container and try to estimate how much the child has swallowed.

**ALLERGENS

BACKGROUND
Allergens are substances that cause allergic reactions in some people. They may be in drugs, plants, animals, the air we breathe, or certain foods.

LEVEL OF DANGER
To an allergic child, even a tiny amount of the allergen can cause serious effects.

SIGNS OF ALLERGIC REACTION (not all signs have to be present)
Symmetric, elevated, and itchy rash on various parts of the body; difficulty in breathing; in severe cases, peeling of skin and mucous membranes, and shock (drop in blood pressure).

WHAT TO DO FOR PREVENTION
For a child with known allergies, consult your physician as to what the child should avoid. For example, children allergic to penicillin are often also allergic to cephalosporine medications. Children allergic to peanuts may endanger their life consuming foods that have even very small amounts of peanuts.

   If the child is known to be seriously allergic, purchase a commercially available kit containing injectable adrenaline, which should be given in case of allergic reaction.

WHAT TO DO IN CASE OF REACTION
1. Give the child an antihistamine tablet or syrup (e.g., Diphenhydramine, Benadryl, or Pheniramine).
2. Take the child to hospital as soon as possible.

****AMITRIPTYLINE

COMMERCIAL NAMES
Adepril, Amitid, Domical, Elavil, Endep, Etrafon, Levate, Levazine, Lumbitrol, Proavil, Triamed, Triavil.

USE
Amitriptyline is an antidepressant medication used mainly for depressive disorders, but also for other psychiatric conditions.

LEVEL OF DANGER
Even one or two tablets can be life-threatening to a small child.

SIGNS OF POISONING (not all signs have to be present)
Unsteadiness; nausea; vomiting; decrease in level of consciousness, shown by drowsiness, sleepiness, unresponsiveness; slow, shallow respiration; grey-blue tinge to skin (cyanosis), which is due to lack of oxygen in blood; cold skin.

  The drug can have life-threatening effects on the heart (changes in rhythm) and on the central nervous system (can cause convulsions or seizures).

WHAT TO DO FOR PREVENTION
If your child is being treated with this drug, be sure to discuss with your physician or pharmacist the exact dose the child needs, the interactions that may occur with other drugs, and side effects of chronic use. Be extremely careful to give the correct dose when switching from liquid to tablets or capsules, and vice versa.

WHAT TO DO IN CASE OF POISONING
1. Remove remaining tablets from mouth.
2. Ensure that the child is breathing and has a heartbeat (see page 3).
3. Induce vomiting with ipecac (see page 5). If the child is sleepy, unconscious, already vomiting, or has had a seizure, do not give ipecac.
4. Take the child to hospital as soon as possible.
5. Bring with you the drug container and try to estimate how much the child has swallowed.

****AMOXAPINE

COMMERCIAL NAMES
Asendin, Demolox, Moxadil, Omnipress.

USE
Amoxapine is an antidepressant medication used mainly for various depressive disorders.

LEVEL OF DANGER
Ingestion of even a few tablets may be life-threatening to a small child.

SIGNS OF POISONING (not all signs have to be present)
Unsteadiness; nausea; vomiting; decrease in level of consciousness, shown by drowsiness, sleepiness, unresponsiveness; slow and/or shallow respiration; grey-blue tinge to skin (cyanosis), which is due to lack of oxygen in blood; cold skin.

The drug can have life-threatening effects on the heart (changes in rhythm) and on the central nervous system (can cause convulsions).

WHAT TO DO IN CASE OF POISONING
1. Remove remaining tablets from mouth.
2. Ensure that the child is breathing and has a pulse (see page 3).
3. Induce vomiting with ipecac (see page 5). If the child is sleepy, unconscious, already vomiting, or has had a seizure, do not give ipecac.
4. Take the child to hospital as soon as possible.
5. Bring with you the drug container and try to estimate how much the child has swallowed.

**ANTIARRHYTHMIC DRUGS

COMMERCIAL NAMES
Biquin, Bretylol, Calan, Cardioquin, Cordarone, Delensol, Deralin, Duraquin, Inderal, Isoptin, Lidocaine, Mexitil, Norpace, Procan, Pronestyl, Propranolol, Prosedyl, Quinaglute Dura-tabs, Quinate, Quivora, Quinidex, Rythmodan, Rythmol, Tambocor, Tonocard.

USE
These drugs are used to treat heartbeat irregularities.

LEVEL OF DANGER
Ingestion by a healthy child is rarely life-threatening, though 300-600 mg of Lidocaine can be very dangerous to a toddler. Children who are treated with antiarrhythmics for heart conditions should be carefully monitored by a specialist, and the parents should be familiar with all potential side effects.

SIGNS OF TOXICITY (not all signs have to be present)
Nausea and vomiting, dizziness, changes in pulse, disappearance of the pulse, and loss of consciousness. Quinidine may cause headache, ringing in the ears, and unsteadiness; Lidocaine may cause convulsions. Because this group has many drugs, read carefully the specific product information sheet to be aware of any additional side effects.

WHAT TO DO FOR PREVENTION
If your child is being treated with antiarrhythmic drugs, be sure to discuss with your physician and pharmacist the exact dose the child needs, the interactions that may occur with other drugs, and side effects of chronic use. Be extremely careful to give the correct dose when switching from liquid to tablets or capsules, and vice versa.

WHAT TO DO IN CASE OF POISONING
1. Remove remaining tablets from mouth.
2. Ensure that the child is breathing and has a heartbeat (see page 3).
3. Induce vomiting with ipecac (see page 5). If the child is sleepy,

unconscious, already vomiting, or has had a seizure, do not give ipecac.
4. Take the child to hospital as soon as possible.
5. Bring with you the drug container, and try to estimate how much the child has swallowed.

*ANTIBIOTICS

GENERIC AND COMMERCIAL NAMES
Achromycin, Amoxil, Ampicillin, Ancef, Anspor, Ceclor, Cefadyl, Cifizox, Chloromycetin, Doxycycline, Erythrocin, Erythromycin, Keflex, Pediazole, Penicillin, Terramycin, Tetracycline, Velosef, Vibramycin, Clavulin, Orbenin, Penbritin, Bactrim, Septra, Trisulfaminic.

USE
Antibiotics are used to treat infections caused by bacteria.

LEVEL OF DANGER
Even in large doses, antibiotics are rarely life-threatening. But if the child is allergic to a specific group of antibiotics, even a very small amount can be life-threatening.

SIGNS OF POISONING (not all signs have to be present)
Nausea, vomiting, and diarrhea after relatively large doses. Signs of allergic reaction are pallor; grey-blue tinge to skin (cyanosis), which is due to lack of oxygen in blood; rapid heartbeat; difficulty in breathing; and changes in consciousness, shown by sleepiness and unresponsiveness; skin rash; and swelling of face, eyes, fingers or other body parts. Because this group of drugs is very large, read the specific product information sheet carefully to be aware of any additional side effects.

WHAT TO DO FOR PREVENTION
If your child is being treated with antibiotics, be sure to discuss with your physician or pharmacist the exact dose the child needs, the interactions that may occur with other drugs, and side effects of chronic use. Be extremely careful to give the correct dose when switching from liquid to tablets or capsules, and vice versa.

WHAT TO DO IN CASE OF POISONING
1. Remove remaining tablets or liquid from mouth.
2. Ensure that the child is breathing and has a heartbeat (see page 3).
3. Induce vomiting with ipecac (see page 5). If the child is sleepy,

unconscious, already vomiting, or has had a seizure, do not give ipecac.
4. Take the child to hospital as soon as possible.
5. Bring with you the drug container, and try to estimate how much the child has swallowed.

**ANTICANCER DRUGS

COMMERCIAL NAMES
Adriamycin, Bienoxane, Cerubidine, Cytosar, Cytoxan, Hydrea, Methotrexate, Mexate, Mithracin, Myleran, Nalulan, Nolvadex, Purinethal, Tamofen.

USE
Anticancer drugs are used, as their name suggests, to fight cancer, but also against various collagen diseases (e.g., lupus erythematosus), or in organ-transplant patients.

LEVEL OF DANGER
These drugs are rarely life-threatening in a single ingestion by a healthy child. They can, however, be dangerous in children with cancer who receive them continuously. Such children should be closely monitored by their doctors.

SIGNS OF POISONING (not all signs have to be present)
Nausea, vomiting, infections due to suppression of white-blood-cell production, and anaemia due to suppression of red-blood-cell production. Because this group of drugs is large, read carefully the specific product information sheet to be aware of any additional side effects.

WHAT TO DO FOR PREVENTION
If your child is being treated with anticancer drugs, be sure to discuss with your physician and pharmacist the exact dose the child needs, the interactions that may occur with other drugs, and side effects of chronic use. Be extremely careful to give the correct dose when switching from liquid to tablets or capsules, and vice versa.

WHAT TO DO IN CASE OF POISONING
1. Remove remaining tablets from mouth.
2. Ensure that the child is breathing and has a heartbeat (see page 3).
3. Induce vomiting with ipecac (see page 5). If the child is sleepy, unconscious, already vomiting, or has had a seizure, do not give ipecac.

4. Take the child to hospital as soon as possible.
5. Bring with you the drug container and try to estimate how much the child has swallowed.

**ANTICONVULSANTS

COMMERCIAL NAMES
Celontin, Milontin, Mysoline, Petinatin, Zarontin.

USE
In addition to phenytoin (Dilantin), carbamazepine (Tegretol), phenobarbital (Phenaphen), and valproic acid (Depakene), which are discussed separately (see pages 93, 40, 92, and 109, respectively), there are many other medications that are given to treat convulsive disorders and epilepsy. These include: clonazepam (Rivotril), primidone (Apo-Primidone Mysoline), Ethosuximide, and trimethadione to mention a few.

LEVEL OF DANGER
These anticonvulsants may be life-threatening, but not often.

- Primidone: poisoning may occur with 1-2 tablets of 250 mg in a toddler weighing 10 kg (22 lb).
- Ethosuximide: Poisoning may occur with 1-2 tablets in a toddler weighing 10 kg (22 lb).

SIGNS OF POISONING (not all signs have to be present)
Nausea and vomiting; signs of bruising of skin; decrease in level of consciousness, shown by drowsiness, sleepiness, or unresponsiveness; slow, shallow breathing; grey-blue tinge to skin (cyanosis), which is due to lack of oxygen in blood; cold skin. Because this is a large group of drugs, read carefully the specific product information sheet to be aware of any additional side effects.

WHAT TO DO FOR PREVENTION
If your child is being treated with this drug, be sure to discuss with your physician or pharmacist the exact dose the child needs, the interactions that may occur with other drugs, and side effects of chronic use. Be extremely careful to give the correct dose when switching from liquid to tablets, and vice versa.

WHAT TO DO IN CASE OF POISONING
1. Remove remaining tablets from mouth.
2. Ensure that the child is breathing and has a heartbeat (see page 3).

3. Induce vomiting with ipecac (see page 5 for instructions). If the child is sleepy, unconscious, already vomiting, or has had a seizure, do not give ipecac.
4. Take the child to hospital as soon as possible.
5. Bring with you the drug container and try to estimate how much the child has swallowed.

****ANTIDEPRESSANTS

GENERIC AND COMMERCIAL NAMES
Trazodone (Desyrel), trimipramine (Surmontil,) Novo-Tripamine Rhotrimine.

USE
In addition to amitriptyline (page 18), amoxapine (page 19), car-bamazepine (page 40), desipramine (page 50), doxepin (page 56), imipramine (page 70), maprotiline (page 77), and nortriptyline (page 87), which are discussed separately in this book, there are many other antidepressants used to treat various forms of depressive disorders and such symptoms as nerve pain.

LEVEL OF DANGER
Even one tablet of antidepressant may be life-threatening to a toddler.

SIGNS OF POISONING (not all signs have to be present)
Unsteadiness; nausea and vomiting; decrease in level of conscious-ness, shown by drowsiness, sleepiness, or unresponsiveness; slow, shallow respiration, grey-blue tinge to skin (cyanosis), which is due to lack of oxygen in blood; cold skin; increase or decrease of heart rate; seizures, or convulsions.

WHAT TO DO IN CASE OF POISONING
1. Remove remaining tablets from mouth.
2. Ensure that the child is breathing and has a heartbeat (see page 3).
3. Induce vomiting with ipecac (see page 5). If the child is sleepy, unconscious, already vomiting, or has had a seizure, do not give ipecac.
4. Take the child to hospital as soon as possible.
5. Bring with you the drug container and try to estimate how much the child has swallowed.

**ANTIDIARRHEAL PREPARATIONS

COMMERCIAL NAMES
Arco-Lase, Bacid, Coly-Mycin, Diban, Donnagel-MB, Fermacal, Furoxone, Gastrolyte, Imodium, Kao-Con, Kaomycin, Kaopectate, Lomotil, Mitrolan, Parepectolin, Pepto-Bismol, Pomalin.

USE
These compounds prevent or control diarrhea mainly by decreasing the motility (natural movement) of the intestine.

LEVEL OF DANGER
The ingesting of even relatively small amounts of antidiarrheals containing opioids, or narcotics (e.g., Lomotil, Imodium), may be life-threatening to a small child.

SIGNS OF POISONING (not all signs have to be present)
Constipation; decrease in level of consciousness, shown by drowsiness, sleepiness, or unresponsiveness; small pupils (in case of narcotics) or dilated pupils (in case of anticholinergics); slow, shallow respiration; rapid pulse; dryness of skin; confusion and hallucinations, especially from anticholinergic antidiarrheals. Because this group contains many different preparations, read the specific product information sheet to be aware of any additional side effects.

WHAT TO DO FOR PREVENTION
If your child is being treated with antidiarrheal medication, be sure to discuss with your physician or pharmacist the exact dose the child needs, the interactions that may occur with other drugs, and side effects of chronic use. Be extremely careful to give the correct dose when switching from liquid to tablets, or capsules, and vice versa.

WHAT TO DO IN CASE OF POISONING
1. Remove remaining tablets from mouth.
2. Ensure that the child is breathing and has a heartbeat (see page 3).
3. Induce vomiting with ipecac (see page 5). If the child is sleepy,

unconscious, already vomiting, or has had a seizure, do not give ipecac.
4. Take the child to hospital as soon as possible.
5. Bring with you the drug container and try to estimate how much the child has swallowed.

*ANTIHISTAMINES

COMMERCIAL NAMES
Actifed, Ambenyl, Antislene, Atrax, Atrohist, Benadryl, Bromfed, Chlor-Tripolon, Claratin, Codimal, Comhist, Comtrex, Corsym, Deconamine, Dimetane, Dimetapp, Dristan, Drixoral, Durrax, Extendryl, Fedabist, Hismanal, Hispril, Histaspan, Isodor, Kronofed, Multipax, Nolahist, Nolamine, Optimine, Ornade, Panectyl, PBZ, Percogesic, Periactin, Phenergan, Polaramine, Pyribenzamine, Quelidrine, Rondec, Ru-Tuss, Rynatan, Rynatuss, Seldane, Simulin, Sinutab, Sudafed, Tacaryl, Tavist, Teldrin, Temaril, Triaminic, Trinalin, Uistaril, Vimicon.

USE
Antihistamines are widely used to ease the symptoms of allergies and colds. In addition, they prevent vomiting and are often used to alleviate morning sickness.

LEVEL OF DANGER
Antihistamines are rarely life-threatening to children. A small child, weighing about 10 kg (22 lb), would usually have to swallow a large number of antihistamines to suffer serious effects.

SIGNS OF POISONING (not all signs have to be present)
Nausea, vomiting, drowsiness, confusion, dry mouth, dry and warm skin, and rapid pulse. A child may occasionally have hallucinations, tremors, excited behaviour, and convulsions.

WHAT TO DO FOR PREVENTION
If your child is being treated with an antihistamine, be sure to discuss with your physician or pharmacist the exact dose the child needs, the interactions that may occur with other drugs, and side effects of chronic use. Be extremely careful to give the correct dose when switching from liquid to tablets, and vice versa.

WHAT TO DO IN CASE OF POISONING
1. Remove remaining tablets from mouth.
2. Ensure that the child is breathing and has a heartbeat (see page 3).
3. Induce vomiting with ipecac (see page 5). If the child is sleepy,

unconscious, already vomiting, or has had a seizure, do not give ipecac.
4. Take the child to hospital as soon as possible.
5. Bring with you the drug container and try to estimate how much the child has swallowed.

**ANTIHYPERTENSIVE DRUGS

COMMERCIAL NAMES
Adalat, Aldaclor, Aldactazide, Aldactone, Aldomet, Aldoril, Apos-azide, Apresoline, Betaloc, Blocraden, Calan, Capoten, Capozide, Cardizem, Catapres, Combipres, Corgard, Corzide, Declinax, Diupres, Diutensen, Dyazide, Enduronyl, Esimil, Exna, Furose-mide, Hydropres, Hydromox, Hygroton, Inderal, Inderide, Ismelin, Loniten, Lopressor, Metatensin, Minipress, Minizide, Moduret, Naquival, Oreticyl, Procardia, Rauzide, Renses, Salukensin, Seapasil, Sectral Senpasil, Simcomem, Sotacor, Tenomin, Ten-oretic, Tenormin, Timolide, Trasicor, Vasotec, Visken, Zuraxolyn.

USE
These drugs are used to treat high blood pressure (hypertension). Some of them are also used in the treatment of other conditions.

LEVEL OF DANGER
Antihypertensive drugs may cause severe effects on health but are very rarely life-threatening following acute ingestion.

SIGNS OF POISONING (not all signs have to be present)
Decrease in blood pressure and changes in heart rate, which may lead to weakness and decrease in level of consciousness; breathing problems, usually caused by the beta blockers; dehydration and acute changes in blood electrolytes (salts), caused by antihyperten-sive drugs that contain diuretics (drugs to increase urine output).

With continuous use, these drugs can cause many different side effects. Because this group of drugs is large, read the specific product information sheet carefully to be aware of additional side effects.

WHAT TO DO FOR PREVENTION
If your child is being treated with an antihypertensive drug, be sure to discuss with your physician or pharmacist the exact dose the child needs, the interactions that may occur with other drugs, and side effects of chronic use. Be extremely careful to give the correct dose when switching from liquid to tablets or capsules, and vice versa.

WHAT TO DO IN CASE OF POISONING

1. Remove remaining tablets from mouth.
2. Ensure that the child is breathing and has a heartbeat (see page 3).
3. Induce vomiting with ipecac (see page 5). If the child is sleepy, unconscious, already vomiting, or has had a seizure, do not give ipecac.
4. Take the child to hospital as soon as possible.
5. Bring with you the drug container and try to estimate how much the child has swallowed.

****ANTIMALARIALS

COMMERCIAL NAMES
Aralen, Plaquenil Sulfate, Primaquine.

USE
Initially used only to prevent or treat malaria. Today, however, they are widely used against inflammatory diseases, such as rheumatoid arthritis and lupus erythematosus.

LEVEL OF DANGER
A small child weighing 10 kg (22 lb) may die from ingestion of 1-2 tablets of these drugs.

SIGNS OF POISONING (not all signs have to be present)
Ear ringing, blurred vision, confusion, weakness. Quinine, quinacrine, chloroquine, and hydroxychloroquine can cause seizures and disturbances in the heartbeat, effects that are life-threatening.

WHAT TO DO FOR PREVENTION
If your child is being treated with an antimalarial medication, be sure to discuss with your physician or pharmacist the exact dose the child needs, the interactions that may occur with other drugs, and side effects of chronic use. Be extremely careful to give the correct dose when switching from liquid to tablets or capsules, and vice versa.

WHAT TO DO IN CASE OF POISONING
1. Remove remaining tablets from mouth.
2. Ensure that the child is breathing and has a heartbeat (see page 3).
3. Induce vomiting with ipecac (see page 5). If the child is sleepy, unconscious, already vomiting, or has had a seizure, do not give ipecac.
4. Take the child to hospital as soon as possible.
5. Bring with you the drug container and try to estimate how much the child has swallowed.

*ARUM

BACKGROUND
The arum family of plants includes the calla lily, elephant ear, jack-in-the-pulpit, caladium, calocasia, and philodendron. All parts of the plants contain oxalate crystals, which are very irritating. Children most commonly ingest jacks-in-the-pulpit.

LEVEL OF DANGER
These plants do not cause systemic (whole body) reactions, only local reactions, which do not endanger life.

SIGNS OF POISONING (not all signs have to be present)
Irritation, pain, and peeling of the mucous membrane (lining) of the mouth, tongue, and throat; nausea and vomiting, diarrhea; and salivation.

WHAT TO DO IN CASE OF POISONING
1. Remove remaining bits of plant from mouth.
2. Give the child a cold drink, preferably milk. Milk binds the irritating oxalate and decreases its damage.
3. Take the child to be examined in a medical facility.

***ASPIRIN (Acetylsalicylic Acid, or ASA)

COMMERCIAL NAMES
ABC compound, Alka Seltzer, Alpha Phed, Anacin (also used for acetaminophen; check label for active ingredient), Ancasal, Arthrinal, Asasantine, Ascriptin, Aspirin, Astin, Breoprin, Bufferin, Coryphen, Dolprin, Dristan, Easprin, Ecotrin, Empirin, Entrophen, Equagesic, Excedrin, Fiogestic, Fiorinal, Lortab ASA, Midol, Norgesic, Novasen, Phenophen, Riphen, Robaxisal, Salpyron, Soma, Strong, Supac, Supasa, Synalgos, Triaphento, Vanquish, Zorprin, U-Way Cold tablets.

USE
Aspirin is widely used for pain, fever, and various inflammations. It is also used as a blood thinner.

LEVEL OF DANGER
Aspirin can be life-threatening to a small child. Three 325-mg tablets in a toddler weighing 10 kg (22 lb), or six tablets in a 20-kg (45-lb) child, can be dangerous. With children's aspirin, which contains only 80 mg per tablet, the two children would need to ingest 12 and 24 tablets respectively.

SIGNS OF POISONING (not all signs have to be present)
Rapid breathing; burning pain in the mouth, throat, or stomach; sleepiness; ringing in ears; vomiting; sleepiness mixed with restlessness; hearing problems; loss of consciousness; seizures; grey-blue tinge to skin (cyanosis), which is due to lack of oxygen in blood.

WHAT TO DO FOR PREVENTION
If your child is being treated with aspirin, be sure to discuss with your physician or pharmacist the exact dose the child needs, the interactions that may occur with other drugs, and side effects of chronic use. Be extremely careful to give the correct dose when switching from liquid to tablets, and vice versa.

Do not give aspirin to children with chicken pox, colds, or flu, as it may cause Reye's syndrome, with severe damage to the liver.

WHAT TO DO IN CASE OF POISONING

1. Remove remaining tablets from mouth.
2. Ensure that the child is breathing and has a heartbeat (see page 3).
3. Induce vomiting with ipecac (see page 5). If the child is sleepy, unconscious, already vomiting, or has had a seizure, do not give ipecac.
4. If resuscitation is needed (the child is not breathing or there is no heartbeat), see pages 3-4.
5. Take the child to hospital as soon as possible.
6. Bring with you the drug container and try to estimate how much the child has swallowed.

*BATTERIES

USE
Small batteries, in sizes that can be swallowed by children, are used for a variety of electric instruments, toys, and watches. Every year thousands of children swallow batteries.

LEVEL OF DANGER
Batteries are dangerous only if they remain stuck in the gastro-intestinal tract, cause obstruction of the gut, or when their corrosive chemicals leak. Perforation of the gut is rare, but can be life-threatening.

Mercury batteries contain only 5 mg of mercuric oxide, so even when broken are not dangerous.

SIGNS OF POISONING (not all signs have to be present)
Nausea, vomiting, or abdominal pain, if batteries leak or their casing opens in the gut.

WHAT TO DO IN CASE OF POISONING
1. *Do not* try to cause vomiting.
2. Take the child to a doctor. The child should be observed until the batteries are expelled in the stool.

**CARBAMAZEPINE

COMMERCIAL NAMES
Tegretol, Novo-Carbamaz, Apo-Carbamazepine.

USE
Carbamazepine is a widely used drug, mainly for epilepsy, but also for depression and various kinds of nerve pain.

LEVEL OF DANGER
Seven or 8 200-mg tablets in a 10-kg (22-lb) toddler can be life-threatening.

SIGNS OF POISONING (not all signs have to be present)
Decrease in level of consciousness, shown by drowsiness, sleepiness, or unresponsiveness; slow, shallow respiration; grey-blue tinge to skin (cyanosis) due to lack of oxygen in blood; cold skin. Children who take the drug regularly may suffer liver, skin, blood, and other problems, though this is rare. Be sure to ask your physician about those.

WHAT TO DO FOR PREVENTION
If your child is being treated with carbamazepine, be sure to discuss with your physician or pharmacist the exact dose the child needs, what interactions may occur with other drugs, and side effects of chronic use. Be extremely careful to give the correct dose when switching from liquid to tablets, or vice versa.

WHAT TO DO IN CASE OF POISONING
1. Remove remaining tablets from mouth.
2. Ensure that the child is breathing and has a heartbeat (see page 3).
3. Induce vomiting with ipecac (see page 5). If the child is sleepy, unconscious, already vomiting, or has had a seizure, do not give ipecac.
4. Take the child to hospital as soon as possible.
5. Bring with you the drug container and try to estimate how much the child has swallowed.

****CARBON MONOXIDE

BACKGROUND
Carbon monoxide is a gas produced by incomplete combustion of fuels, coal, cooking gases, or wood. Commonly, children are poisoned by faulty stoves, heaters, and cars.

LEVEL OF DANGER
Carbon monoxide levels over 100 parts per million of air will cause poisoning in adults, as well as in children. Ideally levels should never be over 9 parts per million. Carbon monoxide causes the death of several children in North America every year.

SIGNS OF POISONING (not all signs have to be present)
Headache, dizziness, rapid pulse, difficulty in breathing, nausea, vomiting, irritability, chest pain, loss of consciousness, pale or bluish skin.

WHAT TO DO IN CASE OF POISONING
1. Open all doors and windows.
2. Remove the child, other people, and animals well away from the poisoned area.
3. Ensure that the child is breathing and has a heartbeat (see page 3).
4. Take the child to hospital as soon as possible.
5. If the child loses consciousness or is not breathing, follow resuscitation procedure as described on page 3.

**CASTOR BEANS (*Ricinus communis*)

BACKGROUND
Castor beans, which contain ricin, a poisonous albumin, are the seeds of the castor-oil plant, which is used for castor oil.

LEVEL OF DANGER
Castor beans can be life-threatening to the child who chews and swallows several.

SIGNS OF POISONING (not all signs have to be present)
Nausea; vomiting; diarrhea; abdominal pain; confusion; grey-blue tinge to skin (cyanosis), which is due to lack of oxygen; loss of consciousness; hemorrhaging in gut; blood in urine; and seizures.

WHAT TO DO IN CASE OF POISONING
1. Remove remaining beans from mouth.
2. Ensure that the child is breathing and has a heartbeat (see page 3).
3. Induce vomiting with ipecac (see page 5). If the child is sleepy, unconscious, already vomiting, or has had a seizure, do not give ipecac.
4. Take the child to hospital as soon as possible.
5. Bring with you a sample of the beans and try to estimate how much the child has swallowed.

***CHLORINATED INSECTICIDES

COMMON INSECTICIDES IN THIS GROUP
Blazer, Amiben, Acarol, Spergon, Quikron, Bidigin, Maintain, Demosan, Jenson, Bravo, Deconil, Tenoran, Rothane, Banvel, Dimilin, Rubigan, Barnon, Suffix BW, Mataven, Flex, Bantrol, Cobra, Topoz, Garlon, Trifmine.

USE
Insecticides are chemicals used to kill insects. This group of insecticides contains chlorinated hydrocarbons such as DDT, Lindane, Benzene hexachloride, and related compounds. While many are now banned (for example, DDT), some, such as Lindane, are widely used.

LEVEL OF DANGER
Chlorinated insecticides may be life-threatening to children. Generally, a dose of .1 g per kg (2 lb) of body weight is highly toxic.

SIGNS OF POISONING (not all signs have to be present)
Nausea, vomiting, nervousness, confusion, dizziness, seizures, loss of consciousness, muscle twitching, tremors.

WHAT TO DO FOR PREVENTION
Lindane should not be used in children for prolonged treatments of scabies or lice.

WHAT TO DO IN CASE OF POISONING
1. Remove remaining chemical from mouth. Wash any areas of child, including eyes, where chemical may have spilled.
2. Ensure that the child is breathing and has a heartbeat (see page 3).
3. Induce vomiting with ipecac (see page 5). If the child is sleepy, unconscious, already vomiting, or has had a seizure, do not give ipecac.
4. Take the child to hospital as soon as possible.
5. Bring with you the chemical and try to estimate how much the child has swallowed.

****CHLORINE GAS

USE
Chlorine is used for water purification, cloth and paper bleaching, and in the manufacture of plastics. In addition, it is used in refrigerators, pharmaceuticals, and cosmetics, to mention a few.

LEVEL OF DANGER
Chlorine is a very corrosive gas. When inhaled, most of the damage is sustained by the respiratory system and may be life-threatening to adults, as well as to children. The danger level is 30 parts per million.

SIGNS OF POISONING (not all signs have to be present)
Coughing, choking, stiffness, headache, increased difficulty in breathing over several hours, chest tightness, and grey-blue tinge to skin (cyanosis), which is due to lack of oxygen in blood.

WHAT TO DO IN CASE OF POISONING
1. Remove the child from the area of exposure.
2. Whether breathing problems appear to exist or not, rush the child to hospital.
3. If the child is not breathing or has lost consciousness, follow resuscitation procedure as described on page 3.

***CODEINE

COMMERCIAL NAMES
ABC, A.C.&C., Acetaco, Codalan, Dimetane, Dolprin, Empracet, G-2, G-3, Naldecon, Novahistex, Nucofed, Pediacof, Penntuss, Percocet, Percodan, Robitussin A-C, Tussar-2, Tussirex.

USE
Codeine, the most widely used narcotic drug, is used to treat moderate to severe pain, such as headaches, toothaches, and so on. It is often abused by individuals addicted to narcotics.

LEVEL OF DANGER
Generally, large doses of codeine tablets are needed to endanger the life of a child. Three 30-mg tablets in a 10-kg (22-lb) toddler can be fatal.

SIGNS OF POISONING (not all signs have to be present)
Unsteadiness; decrease in level of consciousness, shown by drowsiness, sleepiness, or unresponsiveness; slow, shallow breathing; grey-blue tinge to skin (cyanosis) which is due to lack of oxygen in blood; cold skin; weak pulse; muscle twitching; seizures; constipation; small pupils.

WHAT TO DO FOR PREVENTION
If your child is being treated with codeine, be sure to discuss with your physician or pharmacist the exact dose the child needs, the interactions that may occur with other drugs, and side effects of chronic use. Be extremely careful to give the correct dose when switching from liquid to tablets, or vice versa.

WHAT TO DO IN CASE OF POISONING
1. Remove remaining tablets of codeine from mouth.
2. Ensure that the child is breathing and has a heartbeat (see page 3).
3. Induce vomiting with ipecac (see page 5). If the child is sleepy, unconscious, already vomiting, or has had a seizure, do not give ipecac.
4. Take the child to hospital as soon as possible.
5. Bring with you the drug container and try to estimate how much the child has swallowed.

*COSMETICS/PERSONAL CARE

USE
Cosmetics contain a variety of chemicals, including thioglycolates and thioglycerol (cold wave lotion), potassium bromate (cold wave neutralizer), potassium hydroxide (cuticle remover), and barium sulfide (depilatories), to mention a few.

LEVEL OF DANGER
Most household preparations contain little or no amount of toxic ingredients to threaten life. However, be sure to read the label. Call your poison control centre or physician to ensure that the compound is not the rare exception (e.g., alkalis, barium sulfide).

SIGNS OF POISONING (not all signs have to be present)
Bowel irritation, nausea and vomiting, mouth and tongue irritation. If the child has ingested a cuticle remover containing an alkali (potassium hydroxide), see Alkalis. If the child has ingested depilatories containing barium sulfide, she may experience tightness of muscles of face and neck, vomiting, diarrhea, muscle tremors, difficulty in breathing, seizures, and changes in heart rate. Eyelash dye may cause eye irritation.

WHAT TO DO IN CASE OF POISONING
1. Call your poison control centre or physician to verify the safety of the compounds.
2. In case of alkali (e.g., potassium hydroxide), see page 16.
3. If the child has abdominal pain give him milk to drink.

**COUGH AND COLD PREPARATIONS

COMMERCIAL NAMES
Actifed, Ambenyl, Benadryl, Benylin, Bromfed, Calcidrine, Chlortripolon, Chloraseptic, Citra-Forte, Codiclear, Codimal, Comtrex, Congespirin, Coricidin, Corsym, Deconamine, Dilaudid, Dimedrine, Dimetapp, Dristan, Drixoral, Drixtab, Dorcol, Eltor, Entrex, Extendryl, Fedahist, Guaifed, Head & Chest, Histalet, Hycodan, Hycomine, Kronofed, Nafine, Naldecon, Nolamine, Novafed, Novahistex, Novated, Nucofed, Omni-Tuss, Ornade, Ornex, Panaris, Pedia Care, Penntuss, Pima, Polaramine, Propagest, Quelidrine, Robitussin, Robitussin, Sine-Aid, Sinutab, Sudafed, Tessalon, Triaminical, Trinalin, Tussi-Organidin, Tursend, Tussar, Tussionex.

USE
These preparations are used to relieve the symptoms of upper-respiratory-tract infections, such as runny nose and cough. They are mixtures of several medications, such as antihistamines, sympathomimetic decongestants, aspirin or acetaminophen, and codeine.

LEVEL OF DANGER
Cold and cough remedies rarely cause life-threatening poisoning. In general, a small child needs to swallow relatively large amounts of cold remedies to be at risk. For example, a toddler of 10 kg (22 lb) needs to swallow at least 5 tablets of the antihistamine Benadryl to be in danger. However, because these preparations are so widely used, there are reports of fatalities (e.g., from antihistamines, the narcotic codeine, and from some decongestants).

SIGNS OF POISONING (not all signs have to be present)
Drowsiness, dryness of mouth, nausea, dilated pupils, rapid pulse, nausea, urinary retention, disorientation, loss of balance, hallucinations, loss of consciousness, excitement, hot skin, and seizures. Because this group contains many different medications, read the specific product information sheet carefully to be aware of any additional side effects.

WHAT TO DO FOR PREVENTION

If your child is being treated with a cough or cold remedy, be sure to discuss with your physician or pharmacist the exact dose the child needs, the interactions that may occur with other drugs, and side effects of chronic use. Be extremely careful to give the correct dose when switching from liquid to tablets or capsules, and vice versa.

WHAT TO DO IN CASE OF POISONING

1. Remove remaining tablets from mouth.
2. Ensure that the child is breathing and has a heartbeat (see page 3).
3. Induce vomiting with ipecac (see page 5). If the child is sleepy, unconscious, already vomiting, or has had a seizure, do not give ipecac.
4. Take the child to hospital as soon as possible.
5. Bring with you the drug container and try to estimate how much the child has swallowed.

****CYANIDE

BACKGROUND
The seeds of apples, cherries, apricots, plums, and jetberries contain cyanide. Cyanide binds to haemoglobin and does not let oxygen get to cells.

USE
Cyanides are used as fumigants, in the rubber industry, as fertilizers, in metal cleaning, hardening, and refining.

LEVEL OF DANGER
Even small amounts of cyanide-containing solutions can be fatal. Between 5 and 25 seeds of the above fruits cause fatalities in small children. (Only the inner part of the seed is dangerous.)

SIGNS OF POISONING (not all signs have to be present)
Dizziness, rapid breathing, nausea and vomiting, flushing, headache, loss of consciousness, seizures.

WHAT TO DO IN CASE OF POISONING
1. If the child has inhaled cyanide, remove to open area. Be sure not to risk yourself.
2. Remove remaining material from mouth.
3. Ensure that the child is breathing and has a heartbeat (see page 3).
4. Induce vomiting with ipecac (see page 5). If the child is sleepy, unconscious, already vomiting, or has had a seizure, do not give ipecac.
5. Take the child to hospital as soon as possible.
6. Bring with you the consumed agent, and try to estimate how much the child has ingested.

****DESIPRAMINE

COMMERCIAL NAMES
Norpramine, Pertofrane.

USE
Desipramine is an antidepressant medication, used mainly for various depressive disorders, but also for other psychiatric conditions.

LEVEL OF DANGER
Ingestion of even a few tablets may be life-threatening to a small child.

SIGNS OF POISONING (not all signs have to be present):
Unsteadiness; nausea and vomiting; decrease in level of consciousness, shown by drowsiness, sleepiness, unresponsiveness; slow, shallow respiration; grey-blue tinge to skin (cyanosis), which is due to lack of oxygen in blood; cold skin.

The drug can have life-threatening effects on the heart (changes in rhythm) and on the central nervous system (can cause convulsions).

WHAT TO DO IN CASE OF POISONING
1. Remove remaining tablets from mouth.
2. Ensure that the child is breathing and has a heartbeat (see page 3).
3. Induce vomiting with ipecac (see page 5). If the child is sleepy, unconscious, already vomiting, or has had a seizure, do not give ipecac.
4. Take the child to hospital as soon as possible.
5. Bring with you the drug container and try to estimate how much the child has swallowed.

****DIGITALIS

COMMERCIAL NAMES
Crystodigin, Lanoxicaps, Lanoxin, Novodigoxin.

USE
Digitalis drugs, and especially digoxin, the most common among them, are widely used for heart failure and some forms of irregular heartbeat.

LEVEL OF DANGER
Even one adult tablet of digoxin can be life-threatening to a toddler.

SIGNS OF POISONING (not all signs have to be present)
Nausea and vomiting, headache, blurring of sight, diarrhea, confusion, changes in level of consciousness (unresponsiveness, sleepiness), changes in heartbeat.

WHAT TO DO FOR PREVENTION
If your child is being treated with a digitalis drug, be sure to discuss with your physician and pharmacist the exact dose the child needs, the interactions that may occur with other drugs, and side effects of chronic use. Be extremely careful to give the correct dose when switching from liquid to tablets, or vice versa. A child receiving digitalis for a heart condition should be followed carefully by a qualified physician.

WHAT TO DO IN CASE OF POISONING
1. Remove remaining tablets from mouth.
2. Ensure that the child is breathing and has a heartbeat (see page 3).
3. Induce vomiting with ipecac (see page 5). If the child is sleepy, unconscious, already vomiting, or has had a seizure, do not give ipecac.
4. Take the child to hospital as soon as possible.
5. Bring with you the drug container and try to estimate how much the child has swallowed.

**DIGITALIS-PRODUCING PLANTS

TYPES
Oleander, foxglove, and lily of the valley.

BACKGROUND
All plants of the oleander family contain a chemical that acts and leads to poisoning similar to the drug digoxin. Leaves of foxglove contain a different chemical, but with the same action.

LEVEL OF DANGER
Ingestion of large amounts is needed to be life-threatening.

SIGNS OF POISONING (not all signs have to be present)
Nausea, vomiting, blurred vision, changes in heartbeat, cardiac arrest, loss of consciousness.

WHAT TO DO IN CASE OF POISONING
1. Remove remaining bits of plant from the child's mouth.
2. Ensure that the child is breathing and has a heartbeat (see page 3).
3. Induce vomiting with ipecac (see page 5). If the child is sleepy, unconscious, already vomiting, or has had a seizure, do not give ipecac.
4. Take the child to hospital as soon as possible.
5. Bring with you a sample and try to estimate how much the child has swallowed.

**DIOXIN

USE
Dioxin and related materials (2,4-dichlorophenoxyacetic acid) are used as pesticides or herbicides.

LEVEL OF DANGER
Dioxin and related compounds can be life-threatening to a child at a dose of 10 mg per kg (2.2 lb) of body weight.

SIGNS OF POISONING (not all signs have to be present)
Burning and pain in mouth, tongue, throat and stomach; nausea and vomiting, muscle soreness, fever, sleepiness, weakness, seizures, and changes in heartbeat. Days to weeks after ingestion the child may have pustules (pimple-like lesions on skin).

WHAT TO DO IN CASE OF POISONING
1. Remove remaining chemical from mouth.
2. Ensure that the child is breathing and has a heartbeat (see page 3).
3. Induce vomiting with ipecac (see page 5). If the child is sleepy, unconscious, already vomiting, or has had a seizure, do not give ipecac.
4. Take the child to hospital as soon as possible.
5. Bring with you the chemical container and try to estimate how much the child has swallowed.

*DIURETICS

COMMERCIAL NAMES
Aldactazide, Aldactone, Aquatensen, Bumex, Capozide, Chlorthalidone, Corzide, Diamox, Diucardin, Diulo, Diuril, Diurtensen, Dureticyl, Dyazide, Dyrenium, Dyreinium, Edecrin, Enduron, Enduronyl, Esidrix, Furosemide, HydroDiuril, Hydromox, Hypoton, Lasix, Lozol, Maxzide, Midamor, Moduretic, Moduret, Naqua, Naturetin, Rauzide, Renese, Saluron, Serparal, Sincomen, Spinonolactone, Thalitone, Timolide, Underile, Viskazide, Zuroxolyn.

USE
As drugs that increase the production of urine, diuretics are given to people who do not produce enough urine or to those who have accumulation of fluids in their body, such as in congestive heart failure or nephrotic syndrome.

LEVEL OF DANGER
Diuretics are rarely life-threatening to healthy small children. However, children who take them regularly for heart or kidney disease must be closely monitored by a physician.

SIGNS OF POISONING (not all signs have to be present)
Large amounts of urine, decrease in blood pressure, dryness of mouth, dehydration, and changes in heart rate due to loss of potassium. Because this group contains many different drugs, read carefully the specific product information sheet to be aware of additional side effects.

WHAT TO DO FOR PREVENTION
If your child is being treated with a diuretic, be sure to discuss with your physician or pharmacist the exact dose the child needs, the interactions that may occur with other drugs, and side effects of chronic use. Be extremely careful to give the correct dose when switching from liquid to tablets, or vice versa.

WHAT TO DO IN CASE OF POISONING
1. Remove remaining tablets from mouth.
2. Ensure that the child is breathing and has a heartbeat (see page 3).

3. Induce vomiting with ipecac (see page 5). If the child is sleepy, unconscious, already vomiting, or has a seizure, do not give ipecac.
4. Take the child to hospital as soon as possible.
5. Bring with you the drug container and try to estimate how much the child has swallowed.

****DOXEPIN

COMMERCIAL NAMES
Adapine, Apoval, Curatin, Sinequan, Triadapin.

USE
Doxepin is an antidepressant medication, used mainly for various depressive disorders, but also for other psychiatric conditions.

LEVEL OF DANGER
Ingestion of even one or two tablets can be life-threatening to a small child.

SIGNS OF POISONING (not all signs have to be present)
Unsteadiness; nausea; vomiting; decrease in level of consciousness, shown by drowsiness, sleepiness, or unresponsiveness; slow, shallow respiration; grey-blue tinge to skin (cyanosis), which is due to lack of oxygen in blood; cold skin.

The drug can have life-threatening effects on the heart (changes in rhythm) and on the central nervous system (can cause convulsions).

WHAT TO DO IN CASE OF POISONING
1. Remove remaining tablets from mouth.
2. Ensure that the child is breathing and has a heartbeat (see page 3).
3. Induce vomiting with ipecac (see page 5). If the child is sleepy, unconscious, already vomiting, or has had a seizure, do not give ipecac.
4. Take the child to hospital as soon as possible.
5. Bring with you the drug container and try to estimate how much the child has swallowed.

*DYES

USE

Dyes, which contain aniline, arsenic, benzene, silver nitrate, or organic solvents, are used in many households to paint furniture and walls, and to colour clothes.

LEVEL OF DANGER

Only a very large amount of dye causes life-threatening poisoning.

SIGNS OF POISONING (not all signs have to be present)

- *Aniline*-containing dyes or inks can cause grey-blue tinge to skin (cyanosis), which is due to lack of oxygen in blood; headache, dizziness, tiredness, fall in blood pressure, and loss of consciousness.
- *Arsenic*-containing dyes may cause abdominal pain, nausea and vomiting, watery or bloody diarrhea, and weakness.
- *Silver nitrate*-containing dyes may cause pain and burning of mouth, blackening of skin and mucous membranes or of other areas of contact, diarrhea, weakness, and loss of consciousness.
- *Organic solvents*-containing dyes (e.g., benzene) may cause nausea and vomiting, cough, irritation to the lungs, difficulty in breathing.

WHAT TO DO IN CASE OF POISONING

1. Identify the chemicals in the dyes and follow instructions. If *organic solvents*, see Paints/Strippers, page 89. If *silver nitrate*, see page 101.
2. Have the child drink milk to dilute the local effects.
3. If the dye contains arsenic, induce vomiting with ipecac (see page 5). If the child is sleepy, unconscious, already vomiting, or has had a seizure, do not give ipecac.
4. Call your poison information centre for more details and instructions.

***ETHANOL

USE
We all know ethanol as alcohol, the beverage, but it is also part of many industrial compounds, as well as medicinal preparations.

LEVEL OF DANGER
One mL of ethanol per kg (2.2 lb) of weight can be dangerous for a child.

SIGNS OF POISONING (not all signs have to be present)
Decrease of inhibitions, lack of co-ordination, slowed reaction time, slurred speech, depression of the central nervous system, sleepiness, loss of consciousness. Small children may experience severe decrease in blood sugar (hypoglycaemia), which may be life-threatening.

WHAT TO DO IN CASE OF POISONING
1. Remove remaining alcohol from mouth.
2. Ensure that the child is breathing and has a heartbeat (see page 3).
3. Induce vomiting with ipecac (see page 5). If the child is sleepy, unconscious, already vomiting, or has had a seizure, do not give ipecac.
4. Give the child a beverage containing a high level of sugar (e.g. sweetened tea, soft drinks).
5. Take the child to hospital as soon as possible.
6. Bring with you a sample of the alcohol in its container and try to estimate how much the child has swallowed.

***ETHYLENE GLYCOL

USE
Ethylene glycol is part of a variety of industrial compounds. It is used as an antifreeze, preservative, and coolant.

LEVEL OF DANGER
One g per kg (2.2 lb) of body weight can be fatal to a child.

SIGNS OF TOXICITY (not all signs have to be present)
Very similar to alcohol (ethanol) intoxication with decreased inhibitions, lack of co-ordination, slurred speech, depression of the central nervous system, loss of consciousness. Here, however, vomiting, headache, rapid breathing, rapid pulse, lack of production of urine, and seizures reflect the much more severe nature of the poisoning.

WHAT TO DO IN CASE OF POISONING
1. Remove remaining material from mouth.
2. Ensure that the child is breathing and has a heartbeat (see page 3).
3. Induce vomiting with ipecac (see page 5). If the child is sleepy, unconscious, already vomiting, or has had a seizure, do not give ipecac.
4. Take the child to hospital as soon as possible.
5. Bring with you the material and its container, and try to estimate how much the child has swallowed.

Ethanol (alcohol) prevents the conversion of ethylene glycol into its toxic form. Therefore, if you are absolutely sure the child has ingested ethylene glycol, consider giving him a little wine, which is about 10% alcohol. For a 15-kg (30–35-lb) child, 100 mL (about ½ cup) is a good amount. Be aware of the fact, however, that wine may increase sleepiness. Consult a physician or your poison control centre before giving the alcohol.

**FAVA BEANS (*Vicia faba*)

BACKGROUND
Many people eat fava beans, but for those who lack the enzyme glucose 6-phosphate dehydrogenase (G-6-PD) in their red blood cells, eating or even inhaling fava pollens can destroy red blood cells.

LEVEL OF DANGER
For children deficient in G-6-PD enzyme, fava can be life-threatening. Adults and children with this deficiency should avoid them, as well as certain common drugs that have a similar effect (see list below).

SIGNS OF POISONING (not all signs have to be present)
Fever, weakness, yellow skin due to jaundice, dark urine, small amount of urine.

WHAT TO DO FOR PREVENTION
1. Never serve fava beans to infants.
2. If your family is known to have G-6-PD deficiency, avoid fava and the list of drugs below altogether.

WHAT TO DO IN CASE OF POISONING
1. Remove remaining beans from the mouth.
2. Ensure that the child is breathing and has a heartbeat (see page 3).
3. Induce vomiting with ipecac (see page 5). If the child is sleepy, unconscious, already vomiting, or has had a seizure, do not give ipecac.
4. Take the child to hospital as soon as possible.
5. Bring with you a sample of the beans and try to estimate how much the child has eaten.

COMMON DRUGS THAT CAN CAUSE HAEMOLYSIS (damage to red blood cells) in children and adults with G-6-PD deficiency
Nalidixic Acid (Negram)
Nitrofurantoin (Furadantin)
Primaquine
Sulfonamides
Dapsone
Chloramphenicol

*****FOOD POISONING

BACKGROUND
Food can be contaminated by various bacteria that either affect the function of the gut or can have general effects on the whole body.

LEVEL OF DANGER
Perhaps the most dangerous form of food poisoning is botulism, caused by the bacteria *Clostridium botulinum,* which excrete a poison, or toxin. Botulism can be fatal to both adults and children. Most other bacterial food poisonings are not dangerous if the child is treated by a doctor. For this reason the degree of danger varies widely.

SIGNS OF POISONING (not all signs have to be present)
Botulism: The bacteria *Clostridium botulinum* grow in underprocessed nonacidic canned food, mainly meats, fish, vegetables, olives and fruits, and honey fruits. Botulism causes paralysis approximately 8 hours after contaminated food is eaten. The first signs are nausea, vomiting, stomach pain, and diarrhea, followed by muscle weakness, blurred speech, double vision, and paralysis of various muscles. If left untreated, victim suffers paralysis of respiration, then death.

Other bacterial food poisoning: Various harmful bacteria grow in various foods. If ingested, the results are nausea, vomiting, stomach cramps, and diarrhea. These occur in 1-6 hrs with *Staphylococcus,* in 8-22 hours with *Clostridium perfringens,* in 1-16 hours with *Bacillus cereus,* and 4-96 hrs after ingestion of *Vibrio parahaemolyticus.* Most of these infections are self-limiting, and last one to several days.

WHAT TO DO FOR PREVENTION
Botulinum toxin is destroyed when boiled for one min, or kept at 80°C (175°F) for 10 min. Boiling does *not* destroy *Staphylococcus* toxin, whereas it will destroy the *Vibria* and *Bacillus* toxins.

Do not leave cooked food at room temperature. After cooking, unconsumed food should be immediately frozen or discarded, before growth of bacteria takes place.

WHAT TO DO IN CASE OF POISONING

If a child shows signs of food poisoning, take him to the doctor. *Hydration* is the most important element of therapy. Let the child drink as much as possible. If he produces urine in regular amounts, his hydration (i.e., amount of fluid in the body) is probably all right. Do not worry about what the child prefers to drink. Soft drinks and fruit juices are fine — all are more than 99% water. Too many parents try to shove into toddlers herbal teas and other drinks that toddlers hate, and so hydration is not achieved. If the child does not keep the drink down and has persistent vomiting, contact your physician again.

**FOREIGN OBJECTS

BACKGROUND
Small children are forever putting things into their mouths — and often swallow them. Sometimes they may inhale them into their lungs (e.g., peanuts).

LEVEL OF DANGER
Sharp objects can get stuck in the throat or esophagus. If stuck in the windpipe, they are life-threatening.

SIGNS OF FOREIGN BODY (not all signs have to be present)
Difficulty in swallowing, pain in the throat or chest, difficulty in breathing, change in skin colour, choking.

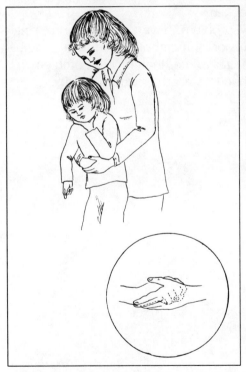

Figure 3. The Heimlich procedure can be used to dislodge such obstructions of the throat as food, toys, or tablets. Stand or kneel behind the child. Close your fist and put the thumb side against the child's belly just below the rib cage. Grasp the fist with your other hand and press up into the belly four times. The pressure should force the obstruction out of the throat.

WHAT TO DO FOR PREVENTION
Never leave a child younger than 6 years of age with peanuts, nuts, or similar foods. These foods are common foreign objects, and after

being crushed in the child's mouth, they are often impossible to remove from the windpipe or lungs.

WHAT TO DO IN CASE OF INGESTION
1. If the child chokes or breathes heavily after swallowing a foreign body, try the Heimlich procedure, which is aimed at releasing a foreign body in the throat. Put your hands together as shown in Figure 3, with the thumb side on the child's upper stomach, just below the middle of the rib cage. Grasp your fist with the other hand. Then press with quick, upward thrusts. Repeat if not successful. This procedure creates high pressure of air in the abdomen and is often strong enough to push the foreign body back into the mouth.
2. *Do not* do the Heimlich procedure if the child is able to speak or whisper, because this means that the larynx (upper part of the windpipe) is not blocked.
3. If there is no breathing problem, have the child drink small amounts of water, milk, or non-carbonated drinks to see if obstruction of the upper gastrointestinal tract is a problem.
4. In any case, rush the child to a nearby medical facility.

***GASES

BACKGROUND
Sometimes a child or the whole family may be exposed to an unknown gas.

LEVEL OF DANGER
Many gases may pose dangers upon inhalation, especially in a closed area. They can be life-threatening.

SIGNS OF POISONING (not all signs have to be present)
Some gases cause irritation of the eyes, nose, and throat, with tearing, coughing, and choking. Other gases are not irritating but affect breathing, causing shortness of breath.

WHAT TO DO IN CASE OF POISONING
1. Remove the child from the exposed area.
2. If the child does not breathe or loses consciousness, follow the resuscitation procedure as described on page 3.
3. Rush the child to nearest medical facility.

***GUN-BLUING COMPOUNDS

BACKGROUND
As name suggests, these compounds, containing selenium, are used in maintenance of guns.

LEVEL OF DANGER
Even small doses taken by the mouth can kill a toddler. Gun-bluing solutions contain lethal amounts of selenium. Ingestion of 15 mL of gun blue by a two-year-old child can be fatal.

SIGNS OF POISONING (not all signs have to be present)
Severe irritation of mouth, throat, gut, difficulty in breathing (after inhalation of fumes), seizures, chills, fever, headaches, respiratory depression, and low blood pressure.

WHAT TO DO IN CASE OF POISONING
1. Ensure that the child is breathing and has a heartbeat (see page 3).
2. Because the compound is a corrosive acid, causing vomiting may increase the damage to the esophagus. On the other hand, the systemic, life-threatening poisoning may lead the physician to induce vomiting. This depends on the amount ingested, if there was spontaneous vomiting, and the condition of the child. There is no antidote for selenium.
3. Have the child drink milk or water (1-3 glasses).
4. Take the child to hospital as soon as possible.
5. Bring with you the remaining gun-bluing compound and try to estimate how much the child has swallowed.

****HEMLOCK (Parsley family)

BACKGROUND
Some plants of the parsley family are poisonous. These include poison hemlock, water hemlock, and dog parsley. They grow along moist areas, such as streams and springs. All parts are poisonous, but the root is the most toxic.

LEVEL OF DANGER
Even a 1-cm piece of water hemlock is life-threatening to a child.

SIGNS OF POISONING (not all signs have to be present):

- *Cicata* — abdominal pain, nausea and vomiting, diarrhea, and vomiting of blood.
- *Conium and dog parsley* — nausea, vomiting, fever, salivation, weakness, paralysis, and respiratory difficulties.

WHAT TO DO IN CASE OF POISONING
1. Remove remaining bits of plant from mouth.
2. Ensure that the child is breathing and has a heartbeat (see page 3).
3. Induce vomiting with ipecac (see page 5). If the child is sleepy, unconscious, already vomiting, or has had a seizure, do not give ipecac.
4. Take the child to hospital as soon as possible.
5. Bring with you sample of the plant and try to estimate how much the child has swallowed.

****HYDROGEN SULPHIDE

USE
This gas, which smells like rotten eggs, is released in various industries, such as the petroleum industry, tanning, rubber, and heavy-water production, but also in sewers.

LEVEL OF DANGER
Level of 50 parts per million of air is dangerous. At that level the odour is pervasive. After a while the smell diminishes as the nose "gets used to it," and the person may be dangerously exposed without being aware. Exposure to hydrogen sulphide can be life-threatening.

SIGNS OF POISONING (not all signs have to be present)
Irritation of eyes, headache, nausea, vomiting, irritation of throat, cough, dizziness, shortness of breathing, loss of consciousness.

WHAT TO DO IN CASE OF POISONING
1. Remove the child from area of exposure.
2. If the child does not breathe or loses consciousness, follow resuscitation procedure as explained on page 3.
3. Rush the child to a medical facility.

****HYPOGLYCAEMICS

COMMERCIAL NAMES (antidiabetic preparations)
DiaBeta, Diabenese, Dirrelor, Dymelor, Glucontral, Glucophage, Micronase, Mobenol, Orirase, Talinase.

USE
These drugs are commonly used by people with diabetes mellitus to decrease blood-sugar level.

LEVEL OF DANGER
Even just one tablet can be life-threatening to a small child.

SIGNS OF POISONING (not all signs have to be present)
Drop in blood sugar (hypoglycaemia), which shows as sweating, pallor, nervousness, nausea, vomiting, confusion, loss of consciousness, and seizures.

WHAT TO DO IN CASE OF POISONING
1. Remove remaining tablets from mouth.
2. Ensure that the child is breathing and has a heartbeat (see page 3).
3. Induce vomiting with ipecac (see page 5). If the child is sleepy, unconscious, already vomiting, or has had a seizure, do not give ipecac.
4. Give the child sugar-containing fluids to drink, which will combat the potential effects of the drug.
5. Take the child to hospital as soon as possible.
6. Bring with you the drug container and try to estimate how much the child has swallowed.

****IMIPRAMINE

COMMERCIAL NAMES
Imipril, Melipamin, Presamine, Tofranil.

USE
Imipramine is used mainly as an antidepressant medication for various depressive disorders. It is also used for children to prevent bed wetting.

LEVEL OF DANGER
Ingestion of even one or two adult tablets can be life-threatening for a small child.

SIGNS OF POISONING (not all signs have to be present)
Unsteadiness; nausea; vomiting; decrease in level of consciousness, shown by drowsiness, sleepiness, or unresponsiveness; slow, shallow respiration; grey-bluish tinge to skin (cyanosis), which is due to lack of oxygen in blood; cold skin.

The drug can have life-threatening effects on the heart (changes in rhythm) and on the central nervous system (can cause convulsions).

WHAT TO DO FOR PREVENTION
If your child is being treated with imipramine, be sure to discuss with your physician or pharmacist the exact dose the child needs, the interactions that may occur with other drugs, and side effects of chronic use. Be extremely careful to give the correct dose when switching from liquids to tablets, or vice versa.

WHAT TO DO IN CASE OF POISONING
1. Remove remaining tablets from mouth.
2. Ensure that the child is breathing and has a heartbeat (see page 3).
3. Induce vomiting with ipecac (see page 5). If the child is sleepy, unconscious, already vomiting, or has had a seizure, do not give ipecac.
4. Take the child to hospital as soon as possible.
5. Bring with you the drug container and try to estimate how much the child has swallowed.

****IRON PREPARATIONS

COMMERCIAL NAMES
Advance, Albafant, Ascofer, Beminal Stress, Calfrate, Cerevon, Ferancee, Fergon, Feritrinsic, Fero-Folic, Fero-Grod, Geurabon, Haematic, Hemocyte Plus, Heptuma Plus, Iberet, Incremin, Iromin, Irospan, Malema, Maltlevol, Mevanin, Niferex, Nu-Iron, Orifer, Orinef, Palafer, Perihemin, Peritinic, Prenate, Prenavite, Pronemia, Poly-Vi-Sol, Slow-Fe, Stresstab, Tropheron.

USE
Iron is needed to build haemoglobin, which gives blood its red appearance. Iron preparations are commonly given to children and adults with iron deficiency anaemia.

LEVEL OF DANGER
The ingestion of iron pills is the leading cause of fatal poisoning in children. Many iron pills look like candies, which of course appeal to small children, who can die from several adult tablets.

SIGNS OF POISONING (not all signs have to be present)
Nausea and vomiting, abdominal pain, dark stools, diarrhea, rapid pulse, low blood pressure, dehydration, and loss of consciousness. These signs may disappear for 24 hours, after which the child may suffer severe cyanosis (grey-blue tinge to skin due to lack of oxygen), breathing difficulties, and loss of consciousness.

WHAT TO DO FOR PREVENTION
If your child is being treated with this drug, be sure to discuss with your physician and pharmacist the exact dose the child needs, the interactions that may occur with other drugs, and side effects of chronic use. Be extremely careful to give the correct dose when switching from liquid to tablets or capsules, and vice versa. If you are pregnant and use iron pills, be sure to keep them out of reach, in a child-proof container.

WHAT TO DO IN CASE OF POISONING
1. Remove remaining tablets from mouth.
2. Ensure that the child is breathing and has a heartbeat (see page 3).

3. Induce vomiting with ipecac (see page 5). If the child is sleepy, unconscious, already vomiting, or has had a seizure, do not give ipecac.
4. Take the child to hospital as soon as possible.
5. Bring with you the drug container and try to estimate how much the child has swallowed.

**ISONIAZID

COMMERCIAL NAMES
INH, Rifamate (includes not only isoniazid), antituberculosis drugs.

USE
Isoniazid is used in the treatment of tuberculosis.

LEVEL OF DANGER
One 300-mg tablet in a 10-kg (22-lb) toddler can be life-threatening.

SIGNS OF POISONING (not all signs have to be present)
Nausea and vomiting, sleepiness, restlessness, confusion, strange behaviour, twitching of muscles, urinary retention, convulsions, and loss of consciousness.

WHAT TO DO FOR PREVENTION
If your child is being treated with isoniazid, be sure to discuss with your physician and pharmacist the exact dose the child needs, the interactions that may occur with other drugs, and side effects of chronic use. Be extremely careful to give the correct dose when switching from liquid to tablets or capsules, and vice versa.

Ensure that the child receives pyridoxine if he is being treated for tuberculosis with isoniazid.

WHAT TO DO IN CASE OF POISONING
1. Remove remaining tablets from mouth.
2. Ensure that the child is breathing and has a heartbeat (see page 3).
3. Induce vomiting with ipecac (see page 5). If the child is sleepy, unconscious, already vomiting, or has had a seizure, do not give ipecac.
4. Take the child to hospital as soon as possible.
5. Bring with you the drug container and try to estimate how much the child has swallowed.

**LEAD

BACKGROUND
Lead is in many things, such as gasoline, batteries, and old paints. Common causes of lead poisoning are battery burning, bullet retention, ceramic glazing, use of unfired pottery, soldering, use of leaden pots, home-distilled whisky/wine, and certain herbal medicines and cosmetics.

LEVEL OF DANGER
A toddler can become very toxic from ingesting a chip of lead paint peeled from a wall. Children rarely die from lead, but many sustain permanent brain damage from chronic exposure.

SIGNS OF POISONING (not all signs have to be present)
Abdominal pain, vomiting, diarrhea, black stools, loss of consciousness, anaemia, problems in concentration and learning, developmental delay, loss of appetite, weight loss, mood swings, and tiredness.

WHAT TO DO FOR PREVENTION
Make sure that your house does not have paints — on walls, furniture, etc. — from before 1940. If it does, then make sure there are no places where paint is peeling, which a child might be tempted to play with and eat.

WHAT TO DO IN CASE OF POISONING
1. Clear the child's mouth.
2. Ensure that the child is breathing and has a heartbeat (see page 3).
3. Induce vomiting with ipecac (see page 5). If the child is sleepy, unconscious, already vomiting, or has had a seizure, do not give ipecac.
4. Take the child to hospital as soon as possible.
5. Bring with you the chemical and try to estimate how much the child has swallowed.

**LITHIUM

COMMERCIAL NAMES
Camcolit, Duralith, Eskalith, Hypnorex, Limas, Lithane, Lithizine, Lithobid, Lithonate.

USE
Lithium is used to treat manic-depressive disorders.

LEVEL OF DANGER
Lithium is rarely life-threatening to a child but it may have serious effects on health. Two 300-mg tablets of lithium carbonate can cause severe toxicity in a 10-kg (22-lb) toddler.

SIGNS OF POISONING (not all signs have to be present)
Nausea; vomiting; diarrhea; change in level of consciousness, shown by drowsiness, or unresponsiveness; unsteadiness; slurred speech; involuntary movements; skin rashes.

WHAT TO DO IN CASE OF POISONING
1. Remove remaining tablets from mouth.
2. Ensure that the child is breathing and has a heartbeat (see page 3).
3. Induce vomiting with ipecac (see page 5). If the child is sleepy, unconscious, already vomiting, or has had a seizure, do not give ipecac.
4. Take the child to hospital as soon as possible.
5. Bring with you the drug container and try to estimate how much lithium the child has swallowed.

**LOCAL ANAESTHETICS

COMMERCIAL NAMES
Analpram, Anbesol, Anestacon, Cetacaine, Corticaine, Dermo-plast Epifoam, Hurricaine, Lidocaine, Lubraseptic, Nupercainal, Pramosone, Proctofoam, Xylocaine.

USE
Local anaesthics are used widely by physicians to prevent pain during certain kinds of surgery. They are also widely used in ointments to treat painful skin or mucous lesions.

LEVEL OF DANGER
Local anaesthetics can be life-threatening to children. One toddler who ingested 300-600 mg of lidocaine had seizures and respiratory difficulties.

SIGNS OF POISONING (not all signs have to be present)
Tremors; seizures, dizziness, unconsciousness; grey-blue tinge to skin (cyanosis), which is due to lack of oxygen in the blood; shallow breathing.

WHAT TO DO IN CASE OF POISONING
1. Remove remaining material from mouth.
2. Ensure that the child is breathing and has a heartbeat (see page 3).
3. Induce vomiting with ipecac (see page 5). If the child is sleepy, unconscious, already vomiting, or has had a seizure, do not give ipecac.
4. Take the child to hospital as soon as possible.
5. Bring with you the drug container and try to estimate how much the child has taken.

****MAPROTILINE

COMMERCIAL NAMES
Ludiomil.

USE
Maprotiline is an antidepressant medication, used in the treatment of various depressive disorders.

LEVEL OF DANGER
Ingestion of even one or two tablets can be life-threatening to a small child.

SIGNS OF POISONING (not all signs have to be present)
Unsteadiness; nausea; vomiting; decrease in level of consciousness, shown by drowsiness, sleepiness, or unresponsiveness; slow, shallow respiration; grey-blue tinge to skin (cyanosis), which is due to lack of oxygen; and cold skin.

The drug can have life-threatening effects on the heart (changes in rhythm) and on the central nervous system (can cause convulsions).

WHAT TO DO IN CASE OF POISONING
1. Remove remaining tablets from mouth.
2. Ensure that the child is breathing and has a heartbeat (see page 3).
3. Induce vomiting with ipecac (see page 5). If the child is sleepy, unconscious, already vomiting, or has had seizures, do not give ipecac.
4. Take the child to hospital as soon as possible.
5. Bring with you the drug container and try to estimate how much the child has swallowed.

*METALLIC MERCURY

USE
Thermometers containing metallic mercury are the most common means of measuring body temperature. Small children often bite the thermometer when their temperature is measured by mouth. Many of them swallow the mercury.

LEVEL OF DANGER
The mercury in thermometers is *not* dangerous to children, because it is not absorbed from the gut into the blood.

SIGNS OF POISONING (not all signs have to be present)
None from toxicity. The child may be traumatized, however, by the glass of the thermometer.

WHAT TO DO IN CASE OF POISONING
Be sure that the child does not have pieces of glass remaining in the mouth. No treatment for the swallowed mercury is needed. (Only mercurial salts and organic mercury are toxic, but they are not part of a thermometer.)

***METALS

USE
Heavy metals, mainly in the form of their salts, are used in numerous industrial compounds.

LEVEL OF DANGER
Ingestion of various solutions of metals can be life-threatening to a child.

SIGNS OF POISONING (not all signs have to be present)
Acute poisoning (e.g., arsenic, cadmium, chromium, lead, mercury) is often characterized by nausea, vomiting, and weakness. Inhalation of some metallic fumes (e.g., beryllium, cadmium, chromium, manganese, mercury) can damage the respiratory system with varying degrees of shortness of breath. Chronic exposure to some metals (e.g., lead, mercury, arsenic, and manganese) can damage peripheral nerves, resulting in a loss of muscle power of sensation, or brain damage.

WHAT TO DO AFTER ACUTE EXPOSURE
1. Remove remaining chemical from mouth.
2. Wash with a large amount of water any area of the child's body where the chemical has spilled.
3. Ensure that the child is breathing and has a heartbeat (see page 3).
4. Induce vomiting with ipecac (see page 5). If the child is sleepy, unconscious, already vomiting, or has had a seizure, do not give ipecac.
5. Take the child to hospital as soon as possible.
6. Bring with you the chemical and try to estimate how much the child has swallowed.

**METHADONE

SOME COMMERCIAL NAMES
Amidon, Dolophine Hydrochloride, Methadone Hydrochloride, Physeptone.

USE
Methadone is a narcotic drug which is used mostly to allow a slow and controlled decrease in the narcotic use of heroin addicts. It is also used to treat severe chronic pain such as in cancer.

LEVEL OF DANGER
Ten mg of methadone can be life-threatening to a child.

SIGNS OF TOXICITY (not all signs have to be present)
Unsteadiness; decreasing level of consciousness, shown by sleepiness or unresponsiveness; slow, shallow breathing, grey-blue tinge to skin (cyanosis), which is due to lack of oxygen; cold skin; weak pulse; muscle twitching; constipation; and small pupils.

WHAT TO DO IN CASE OF POISONING
1. Remove remaining methadone from mouth.
2. Ensure that the child is breathing and has a heartbeat (see page 3).
3. Induce vomiting with ipecac (see page 5). If the child is sleepy, unconscious, already vomiting, or has had a seizure, do not give ipecac.
4. Take the child to hospital as soon as possible.
5. Bring with you the drug container and try to estimate how much the child has swallowed.

*METHANE/NATURAL GAS

USE
A mixture of these gases is commonly used for cooking.

LEVEL OF DANGER
A severe leak of these gases may be life-threatening to a child, but a level of 1000 parts per million of air is usually not dangerous.

SIGNS OF POISONING (not all signs have to be present)
These gases do not irritate the respiratory system, but by depleting the air of oxygen, breathing becomes difficult. Victims may lose consciousness or have cardiac irregularities.

WHAT TO DO IN CASE OF POISONING
1. Remove the child from the area of exposure.
2. Open all doors and windows.
3. If the child is not breathing or loses consciousness, follow resuscitation procedure as explained on page 3.
4. Rush the child to nearest medical facility.

****MORPHINE**

SOME COMMERCIAL NAMES
Epimorph, MS Contin, Roxanal, Statex, MSIR.

USE
Morphine is a narcotic drug. In its tablet form, it is widely used by patients with chronic, severe pain, such as in cancer. It is widely abused and therefore can be found in thousands of households.

LEVEL OF DANGER
As few as two 100-mg tablets of morphine can be life-threatening to a toddler.

SIGNS OF POISONING (not all signs have to be present)
Unsteadiness, decrease in levels of consciousness (i.e., sleepiness, unresponsiveness), slow, shallow breathing, grey-blue skin (cyanosis), which is due to lack of oxygen, cold skin, weak pulse, muscle twitching, constipation, small pinpoint pupils.

WHAT TO DO FOR PREVENTION
If your child is treated with morphine, be sure to discuss with your physician or pharmacist the exact dose the child needs, the interactions that may occur with other drugs, and side effects of chronic use.

WHAT TO DO IN CASE OF POISONING
1. Remove remaining tablets from mouth.
2. Ensure that the child is breathing and has a heartbeat (see page 3).
3. Induce vomiting with ipecac (see page 5). If the child is sleepy, unconscious, already vomiting, or has had a seizure, do not give ipecac.
4. Take the child to hospital as soon as possible.
5. Bring with you the drug container and try to estimate how many tablets the child could have ingested.

**MUSHROOMS

BACKGROUND
There are many edible mushrooms, but a good number are very toxic.

LEVEL OF DANGER
Even one toxic mushroom can be life-threatening to a child.

SIGNS OF POISONING (not all signs have to be present)
Poisoning depends on the mushrooms: nausea and vomiting (almost all toxic mushrooms); diarrhea (mushrooms containing amatoxins and phallotoxins); stomach pain (many different mushrooms); breathing difficulties (muscarine-releasing mushrooms); changes in behaviour and level of consciousness (mushrooms containing indoles); and serious liver damage (amatoxins, phallotoxins).

WHAT TO DO FOR PREVENTION
Never experiment with mushrooms. Eat only mushrooms known to you.

WHAT TO DO IN CASE OF POISONING
1. Remove remaining bits of mushroom from mouth.
2. Ensure that the child is breathing and has a heartbeat (see page 3).
3. Induce vomiting with ipecac (see page 5). If the child is sleepy, unconscious, already vomiting, or has had a seizure, do not give ipecac.
4. Take the child to hospital as soon as possible.
5. Bring with you a sample of the mushroom and try to estimate how much the child could have swallowed.

***NARCOTIC ANALGESICS

COMMERCIAL NAMES
Bancap, Dilaudid, Dionin, Dolophine, Imodium, Leritine, Lomotil, Nisentil, Novrad, Prinadal, Stadal, Talwin.

USE
Many narcotic analgesic drugs are on the market to treat various forms of severe pain. Most of them have similar signs of poisoning, although there is variability that is beyond the scope of this book.

LEVEL OF DANGER
Even relatively small amounts of a narcotic can be life-threatening to children. Here are the fatal doses of some common narcotics:

- Lomotil (diphenoxylate) — 20 2.5-mg tablets killed a 2½-year-old.
- Talwin (pentazocine) — 2 50-mg tablets killed a 2½-year-old.

SIGNS OF POISONING (not all signs have to be present)
Unsteadiness; decrease in level of consciousness, shown by drowsiness, sleepiness, or unresponsiveness; slow, shallow breathing; grey-blue tinge to skin (cyanosis), which is due to lack of oxygen; cold skin; weak pulse; muscle twitching; seizures; constipation; and pinpoint pupils. Narcotic analgesics are often combined with acetaminophen or aspirin, and overdose of these drugs may also happen and should be treated (see pages 11 and 37–38).

WHAT TO DO IN CASE OF POISONING
1. Remove remaining tablets from mouth.
2. Ensure that the child is breathing and has a heartbeat (see page 3).
3. Induce vomiting with ipecac (see page 5). If the child is sleepy, unconscious, already vomiting, or has had a seizure, do not give ipecac.
4. Take the child to hospital as soon as possible.
5. Bring with you the drug container and try to estimate how much the child has swallowed.

**NIGHTSHADE (Solanaceae)

TYPES
Potatoes, tomatoes, and related plants

BACKGROUND
These vegetables contain small amounts of the poison solanine. However, there are larger amounts of the poison in the leaves and the unripened green vegetables. The sprouts, stems, and green skin have the greatest concentration. These vegetables grow all over North America.

LEVEL OF DANGER
In a few instances, consumption of *several* unripe vegetables has resulted in life-threatening signs. Death has occurred only in malnourished, untreated children.

SIGNS OF POISONING (not all signs have to be present)
Seven to 19 hours after consumption: nausea, vomiting, diarrhea, weakness, fever, drowsiness, confusion, delirium, and headache.

WHAT TO DO IN CASE OF POISONING
1. Remove any remaining bits of fruit and leaves from mouth.
2. Ensure that the child is breathing and has a heartbeat (see page 3).
3. Induce vomiting with ipecac (see page 5). If the child is sleepy, unconscious, already vomiting, or has had a seizure, do not give ipecac.
4. Take the child to hospital as soon as possible.
5. Bring with you a plant sample and try to estimate how much the child has swallowed.

*NON-STEROIDAL ANTI-INFLAMMATORY DRUGS (NSAIDs)

COMMERCIAL NAMES
Annox, Clinoril, Dolobid, Feldene, Ibuprofen, Indocin, Medomen, Motrin, Naflon, Naprosyn, Ponstel, Tolectin.

NSAIDs are widely used to combat cold, headache, toothache, migraines, and chronic pain. They are also used to treat inflammatory disease (e.g., rheumatoid arthritis).

LEVEL OF DANGER
A large number of tablets must be ingested to be life-threatening, unless they are mixed with aspirin.

SIGNS OF POISONING (not all signs have to be present)
Nausea, vomiting, stomach pain, headache, and sleepiness.

WHAT TO DO FOR PREVENTION
If your child is treated with an NSAID medication, be sure to discuss with your physician or pharmacist the exact dose the child needs, the interactions that may occur with other drugs, and side effects of chronic use. Be extremely careful to give the correct dose when switching from liquid to tablets, or vice versa.

WHAT TO DO IN CASE OF POISONING
1. Remove remaining tablets from mouth.
2. Ensure that the child is breathing and has a heartbeat (see page 3).
3. Induce vomiting with ipecac (see page 5). If the child is sleepy, unconscious, already vomiting, or has had a seizure, do not give ipecac.
4. Take the child to hospital as soon as possible.
5. Bring with you the drug container and try to estimate how much the child has swallowed.

****NORTRIPTYLINE

COMMERCIAL NAMES
Allergon, Altilev, Auentyl, Pamelor, Vividyl.

USE
Nortriptyline is an antidepressant, used to treat various forms of depression.

LEVEL OF DANGER
Even one or two adult tablets can be life-threatening to a child.

SIGNS OF POISONING (not all signs have to be present)
Unsteadiness; nausea; vomiting; decrease in level of consciousness, shown by drowsiness, sleepiness, or unresponsiveness; slow, shallow respiration; grey-blue tinge to skin (cyanosis), which is due to lack of oxygen in blood; cold skin.

The drug can have life-threatening effects on the heart (changes in rhythm) and on the central nervous system (can cause convulsions).

WHAT TO DO IN CASE OF POISONING
1. Remove remaining tablets from mouth.
2. Ensure that the child is breathing and has a heartbeat (see page 3).
3. Induce vomiting with ipecac (see page 5). If the child is sleepy, unconscious, already vomiting, or has had a seizure, do not give ipecac.
4. Take the child to hospital as soon as possible.
5. Bring with you the drug container and try to estimate how much the child has swallowed.

***ORGANOPHOSPHATE AND CARBAMATE PESTICIDES

COMMERCIAL NAMES
Abate, Acephate, Aldicarb, Bromophos, Butacarb, Carbaryl, Chlormephos, Cyanophos, Diazinon, Dimetan, Guthion, Isocarb, Isophenphos, Malathion, Nexion, Orthene, Parathione, Temophos, Thiodicarb.

USE
These compounds are commonly used to kill insects.

LEVEL OF DANGER
Some organophosphates (e.g., parathione) can be life-threatening to children even following agricultural spraying. Others (e.g., diazinon) are dangerous only upon ingestion of .5 g/kg of weight; e.g., a 10-kg (22-lb) child is endangered by ingesting 5 g.

SIGNS OF POISONING (not all signs have to be present)
Headache, stomach cramps, vomiting, diarrhea, dizziness, weakness, sweating, hot skin, salivation, breathing difficulties, unsteadiness, seizures, slow heart rate, pinpoint pupils, muscle twitching, and paralysis.

WHAT TO DO IN CASE OF POISONING
1. Wash any areas on body where chemical may have had contact. In case of skin exposure by a spray, take off all clothing, wash the child thoroughly while protecting yourself with gloves and a mask.
2. Ensure that the child is breathing and has a heartbeat (see page 3).
3. Induce vomiting with ipecac (see page 5). If the child is sleepy, unconscious, already vomiting, or has had a seizure, do not give ipecac.
4. Take the child to hospital as soon as possible.
5. Bring with you the chemical and try to estimate how much the child has ingested.

*PAINTS/STRIPPERS

BACKGROUND
A variety of oil- and water-based household paints are ingested by children every year.

LEVEL OF DANGER
Most paints and paint strippers are not life-threatening upon ingestion. However, inhalation of the organic solvents (e.g., turpentine) or strippers may cause damage to the lungs.

SIGNS OF POISONING (not all signs have to be present)
Nausea, vomiting, burning of mouth, cough, difficulty in breathing.

WHAT TO DO IN CASE OF POISONING
1. *Do not* try to induce vomiting, because vomiting may cause damaging inhalation of vapours into the lungs.
2. Remove remaining material from mouth.
3. Give the child one or two glasses of milk or water.
4. Wash carefully, using a large amount of water, any areas of the body that paint or solvent may have contacted.
5. Take the child to hospital as soon as possible.
6. Bring with you a sample of the material in its container and try to estimate how much the child has swallowed.

****PARAQUAT

USE
Paraquat is used in agriculture as a herbicide.

LEVEL OF DANGER
Ingestion of even a tiny amount of paraquat solution can kill a child.

SIGNS OF POISONING (not all signs have to be present)
Immediately after ingestion — nausea, vomiting, stomach pain, burning sensation of mouth and throat, tongue. Around a week after exposure — lung damage causes increased shortness of breath and respiratory failure.

WHAT TO DO IN CASE OF POISONING
1. Rinse child's mouth of chemical.
2. Ensure that the child is breathing and has a heartbeat (see page 3).
3. Try to rinse any remaining solution from the child's mouth.
4. Induce vomiting with ipecac (see page 5). If the child is sleepy, unconscious, already vomiting, or has had a seizure, do not give ipecac.
5. Take the child to hospital as soon as possible.
6. Bring with you remaining chemical and try to estimate how much the child has swallowed.

**PETROLEUM PRODUCTS (Hydrocarbons)

USE
Petroleum products contain hydrocarbons, which are widely used as fuels and solvents of numerous chemicals. The common hydrocarbons include: benzene, diesel oil, fuel oil, gasoline, kerosene, lubricating oils, mineral spirit, petroleum, toluene, turpentine, and xylene.

LEVEL OF DANGER
Even a large amount of an ingested, or swallowed, hydrocarbon is relatively nontoxic. On the other hand, inhalation of even a small amount can cause serious lung damage. Often other compounds are dissolved in the solvent (e.g., insecticides, Paraquat), and they may be much more toxic.

SIGNS OF POISONING (not all signs have to be present)
Nausea, vomiting, cough due to irritation of the windpipe and lungs, shortness of breath, sleepiness, weakness, loss of consciousness.

WHAT TO DO IN CASE OF POISONING
1. *Do not* induce vomiting because the returning material may be inhaled and cause damage to the lungs.
2. Identify what chemicals, if any, were dissolved in the organic solvent the child has swallowed. If the organic solvent contains other, more toxic compounds, your poison control centre may instruct you whether induction of vomiting is warranted to avoid the risk of these poisons, despite the risk of inhalation of the hydrocarbons.
3. Take the child to hospital as soon as possible.
4. Bring with you the chemical and try to estimate how much the child has swallowed.

****PHENOBARBITAL**

COMMERCIAL NAMES
Anco-Lase, Antrocal, Azpan, Belianderal, Bellanderal, Gardenal, Gustase Plus, Hyprolone, Luminal, Mediphen, Neurotransentin, Phenaphen, Mudrane, Phazyme, Primatene, Quadrinal, Theofedral.

USE
Phenobarbital is used in the treatment of epilepsy, and its sedative-hypnotic properties induce sleep. Many forms of convulsive disorders in infants and children are treated with this drug.

LEVEL OF DANGER
Phenobarbital can be life-threatening to the overdosed child. Two tablets of Luminal can endanger a 10-kg (22-lb) toddler.

SIGNS OF POISONING (not all signs have to be present)
Drowsiness, headache, sleepiness, slurred speech, unsteadiness, loss of consciousness, constricted pupils, and shallow breathing.

WHAT TO DO FOR PREVENTION
If your child is being treated with phenobarbital, be sure to discuss with your physician or pharmacist the exact dose the child needs, the interactions that may occur with other drugs, and side effects of chronic use. Be extremely careful to give the correct dose when switching from liquid to tablets, or vice versa.

WHAT TO DO IN CASE OF POISONING
1. Remove remaining tablets of phenobarbital from mouth.
2. Ensure that the child is breathing and has a heartbeat (see page 3).
3. Induce vomiting with ipecac (see page 5). If the child is sleepy, unconscious, already vomiting, or has had a seizure, do not give ipecac.
4. Take the child to hospital as soon as possible.
5. Bring with you the drug container and try to estimate how many tablets the child has swallowed.

**PHENYTOIN (Diphenylhydantoin)

COMMERCIAL NAMES
Dilantin.

USE
Phenytoin is widely used to treat epilepsy and other disorders of the central nervous system.

LEVEL OF DANGER
Phenytoin can be life-threatening to a child. Three 100-mg tablets can seriously harm a 10-kg (22-lb) toddler.

SIGNS OF POISONING (not all signs have to be present)
Unsteadiness; nausea; vomiting; decrease in level of consciousness, shown by drowsiness, sleepiness, or unresponsiveness; slow, shallow respiration; grey-blue tinge to skin (cyanosis), which is due to lack of oxygen; and cold skin. Children receiving the drug continuously may experience swelling of gums; liver, kidney, and blood problems; and excessive growth of hair.

WHAT TO DO FOR PREVENTION
If your child is being treated with phenytoin, be sure to discuss with your physician or pharmacist the exact dose the child needs, the interactions that may occur with other drugs, and side effects of chronic use. Be extremely careful to give the correct dose when switching from liquid to tablets, or vice versa.

WHAT TO DO IN CASE OF POISONING
1. Remove remaining tablets from mouth.
2. Ensure that the child is breathing and has a heartbeat (see page 3).
3. Induce vomiting with ipecac (see page 5). If the child is sleepy, unconscious, already vomiting, or has had a seizure, do not give ipecac.
4. Take the child to hospital as soon as possible.
5. Bring with you the drug container and try to estimate how much the child has swallowed.

PLANTS (Type Unknown)

BACKGROUND
Plants are among the most common things children ingest and, therefore, a major source of concern to parents.

LEVEL OF DANGER
Many plants are not poisonous, but some can be life-threatening.

SIGNS OF POISONING (not all signs have to be present)
Stomach pain, nausea, vomiting, and weakness.

WHAT TO DO FOR PREVENTION
1. Become familiar with the names and nature of the plants in your house and garden.
2. Call the poison control centre for specific information on each.

WHAT TO DO IN CASE OF POISONING
1. Call your poison control centre.
2. If you do not know the plant ingested, induce vomiting with ipecac (see page 5) and rush the child to the nearest medical facility.

*POKEWEED (*Phytolacca americana*)

BACKGROUND
All parts of this plant, but especially the root, have toxic chemicals that can irritate the gut.

LEVEL OF DANGER
Pokeweed mainly causes gastroenteritis (inflammation of the lining of stomach and intestines) and does not usually endanger life.

SIGNS OF POISONING (not all signs have to be present)
Irritation and burning of mouth and throat, nausea, vomiting, diarrhea, slow respiratory rate, and weakness.

WHAT TO DO IN CASE OF POISONING
1. Remove any remaining bits of pokeweed from mouth.
2. Give the child milk to drink.
3. Ensure that the child is breathing and has a heartbeat (see page 3).
4. Induce vomiting with ipecac (see page 5). If the child is sleepy, unconscious, already vomiting, or has had a seizure, do not give ipecac.
5. Take the child to hospital as soon as possible.
6. Bring with you the sample of the plant and try to estimate how much the child has ingested.

**PROPOXYPHENE

COMMERCIAL NAMES
Darvocet, Darvon, Propacet.

USE
Propoxyphene is a narcotic drug that is used to treat severe pain. It is widely abused and therefore can be found in thousands of households.

LEVEL OF DANGER
Six 65-mg tablets in a 10-kg (22-lb) toddler can be dangerous, but propoxyphene has rarely been life-threatening to a child.

SIGNS OF POISONING (not all signs have to be present)
Unsteadiness; decrease in level of consciousness, shown by drowsiness, sleepiness, or unresponsiveness; slow, shallow breathing; grey-blue tinge to skin (cyanosis), which is due to lack of oxygen; cold skin; weak pulse; muscle twitching; constipation; and pinpoint pupils.

WHAT TO DO FOR PREVENTION
If your child is being treated with propoxyphene, be sure to discuss with your physician or pharmacist the exact dose the child needs, the interactions that may occur with other drugs, and side effects of chronic use. Be extremely careful to give the correct dose when switching from liquid to tablets, or vice versa.

WHAT TO DO IN CASE OF POISONING
1. Remove remaining tablets from mouth.
2. Ensure that the child is breathing and has a heartbeat (see page 3).
3. Induce vomiting with ipecac (see page 5). If the child is sleepy, unconscious, already vomiting, or has had a seizure, do not give ipecac.
4. Take the child to hospital as soon as possible.
5. Bring with you the drug container and try to estimate how much the child has swallowed.

**RIFAMPIN

COMMERCIAL NAMES
Rifadin, Rifamide, Rimactane, Rofact.

USE
Rifampin is used in the treatment of tuberculosis and to prevent certain forms of bacterial meningitis.

LEVEL OF DANGER
Two 30-mg tablets of rifampin in a 10-kg (22-lb) toddler may be dangerous, but acute ingestion of rifampin is rarely life-threatening.

SIGNS OF POISONING (not all signs have to be present)
Nausea and vomiting, unexplained changes in behaviour, orange-red colour of skin, sleepiness, itching.

WHAT TO DO FOR PREVENTION
If your child is being treated with rifampin, be sure to discuss with your physician and pharmacist the exact dose the child needs, the interactions that may occur with other drugs, and side effects of chronic use. Be extremely careful to give the correct dose when switching from liquid to tablets or capsules, and vice versa.

WHAT TO DO IN CASE OF POISONING
1. Remove remaining tablets from mouth.
2. Ensure that the child is breathing and has a heartbeat (see page 3).
3. Induce vomiting with ipecac (see page 5). If the child is sleepy, unconsciousness, already vomiting, or has had a seizure, do not give ipecac.
4. Take the child to hospital as soon as possible.
5. Bring with you the drug container and try to estimate how much the child has swallowed.

*RHUBARB (*Rheum*)

BACKGROUND
The leafy parts of rhubarb contain the irritating chemical oxalic acid.

LEVEL OF DANGER
Rhubarb is not life-threatening to a healthy child.

SIGNS OF POISONING (not all signs have to be present)
Pain in mouth, drooling, nausea, vomiting, diarrhea, stomach pain, reduced kidney function (less urine), hemorrhaging.

WHAT TO DO IN CASE OF POISONING
1. Remove remaining rhubarb leaves from mouth.
2. Ensure that the child is breathing and has a heartbeat (see page 3).
3. Induce vomiting with ipecac (see page 5). If the child is sleepy, unconscious, already vomiting, or has had a seizure, do not give ipecac.
4. Give the child milk to drink, which precipitates the oxalate poison.
5. Take the child to hospital as soon as possible.
6. Bring with you a plant sample and try to estimate how much the child has swallowed.

**SEDATIVE-HYPNOTIC DRUGS

COMMERCIAL NAMES
Alurate, BAC, Benadryl, Centrex, Cloropin, Dalmane, Equanil, Excedrin, Halcion, Hydroxyzine, Largon, Librium, Mepergan, Mogadone, Nebaral, Nembutal, Noludar, Pentobarbital, Phenergan, Placidyl, Plexonal, Restoril, Sedapap, Serax, Somnal, Tranxene, Tuinal, Unisom Nighttime, Valium, Valmid, Versed, Zanax.

USE
These drugs are widely used to help people fall asleep, to relax them, or to treat stress.

LEVEL OF DANGER
Several tablets of many of these drugs can cause a child to fall into prolonged deep sleep, with little response, but rarely endanger life. The fatal dose for most of the drugs is .1-.5 g/kg of body weight.

SIGNS OF POISONING (not all signs have to be present)
Tiredness; confusion; nervousness; sleepiness; loss of consciousness; slow, shallow breathing; unsteadiness; flaccid muscles; grey-blue tinge to skin (cyanosis), which is due to lack of oxygen; and cold skin. Because this group contains many drugs, read carefully the specific product information sheet to be aware of additional side effects.

WHAT TO DO FOR PREVENTION
If your child is being treated with a sedative-hypnotic medication, be sure to discuss with your physician and pharmacist the exact dose the child needs, the interactions that may occur with other drugs, and side effects of chronic use. Be extremely careful to give the correct dose when switching from liquid to tablets or capsules, and vice versa.

WHAT TO DO IN CASE OF POISONING
1. Remove remaining tablets from mouth.
2. Ensure that the child is breathing and has a heartbeat (see page 3).
3. Induce vomiting with ipecac (see page 5). If the child is sleepy,

unconscious, already vomiting, or has had a seizure, do not give ipecac.
4. Take the child to hospital as soon as possible.
5. Bring with you the drug container and try to estimate how much the child has swallowed.

***SILVER NITRATE

USE
Silver nitrate kills bacteria and is therefore useful as an antiseptic agent for skin and mucous membranes.

LEVEL OF DANGER
Even a small amount (1-2 mL) of the salt can be life-threatening to a small child.

SIGNS OF POISONING (not all signs have to be present)
Blackening of the mouth or other areas of contact on the skin, vomiting, loss of consciousness, pain and burning in the mouth, salivation, vomiting of black content, diarrhea, and seizures.

WHAT TO DO FOR PREVENTION
If your child is being treated with silver nitrate, be sure to discuss with your physician or pharmacist the exact amount the child needs.

WHAT TO DO IN CASE OF POISONING
1. *Do not* induce vomiting, because this dangerous salt will again have contact with the esophagus and mouth.
2. Have the child drink large amounts of water containing regular table salt — 10 gm (2 tsp) of salt per 1 litre (qt) of water.
3. Take the child to hospital as soon as possible.
4. Bring with you the chemical container and try to estimate how much the child has swallowed.

***SNAKE VENOM

BACKGROUND
Most snake bites are not poisonous, but those that are release a venom that is life-threatening. The most common venomous snakes in North America are the copperhead and rattlesnake.

LEVEL OF DANGER
Poisonous snake bites may be life-threatening. Children are in more danger than adults because the poison spreads into a smaller space. If the type of snake is unknown, you should assume it is venomous (poisonous) until proven otherwise.

SIGNS OF POISONING (not all signs have to be present)
Swelling, pain, and skin-colour changes at the site of bite, nausea, vomiting, pallor, weakness, sweating, loss of consciousness, tingling of tongue and mouth, and rapid pulse.

WHAT TO DO FOR PREVENTION
If you live in areas with venomous snakes (e.g., Arizona, Colorado), be sure that your child wears shoes and thick canvas leggings when walking in grassy or busy areas.
   Avoid walking in such areas at night.

WHAT TO DO IN CASE OF POISONING
1. Have child lie down and be still. The child should not walk, because this increases circulation and spreading of the venom.
2. Wash the bitten area with water to remove the poison from the surface. Do not mess with bitten area.
3. Rush the child to a medical facility for antiserum (shots against the venom).
4. If snake has been killed, bring it with you for identification.
5. If symptoms develop quickly while on way to medical facility, a ½ × 24-in rubber band or ⅛-inch diameter thin-walled gum rubber tubing may be applied just above the bitten area (between it and the centre of the body). The band should not be applied too tightly; the idea is to stop only the lymph supply, not the blood supply.

6. Ensure that the child is breathing and has a heartbeat (see page 3).
7. If the child is in pain give her acetaminophen (Tylenol) or acetaminophen with codeine.

***SPIDER AND SCORPION BITES

BACKGROUND
Scorpions are found in Texas, Arizona, New Mexico, California, Nevada, Michigan, and Saskatchewan. Black widow spiders are found in southern and eastern USA. Brown recluse spiders, while found in California, are mainly in southeastern USA.

LEVEL OF DANGER
Even one bite can be life-threatening to a child, especially if it is on the face or neck.

SIGNS OF POISONING (not all signs have to be present)
Severe pain, swelling, skin-colour changes in area of bites, bleeding in area, nausea, vomiting, pallor, weakness, sweating, loss of consciousness, tingling of tongue and mouth, and rapid pulse.

WHAT TO DO FOR PREVENTION
If you live in areas with any of these species, be sure that your child wears shoes, socks, and thick pants when walking in grassy or bushy areas.

Avoid walking in such areas at night.

WHAT TO DO IN CASE OF POISONING
1. Ensure child is breathing and has a heartbeat (see page 3).
2. Have the child lie down and be still. The child should not walk, because walking increases circulation and spreading of the venom.
3. Wash the bitten area with water to remove the poison from the surface. Do not mess with bitten area.
4. Rush the child to a medical facility for antiserum (shots against the venom).
5. If spider or scorpion has been killed, bring it with you for identification.
6. If the child is in pain, give him acetaminophen (Tylenol) or acetaminophen with codeine.

****STREET DRUGS

STREET NAMES
Angel dust (phencyclidine), skag, dope, shill, H, white stuff, Lady Jane (heroin), china white (Lentanyl), snow, Dama Blanca, flake, gold dust, greengold, coke (cocaine), speedball (heroin and cocaine), liquid lady (alcohol and cocaine).

USE
Street drugs, mostly illegal, are used by people to achieve euphoria or relaxation. Some are prescribed medications that are abused. The drug classifications vary widely and, therefore, effects differ substantially.

LEVEL OF DANGER
Even relatively small doses of narcotics, cocaine, phencyclidine (PCP), or LSD can be dangerous to small children. Small children exposed to crack-cocaine smoke may become very sick.

SIGNS OF POISONING (not all signs have to be present):

- **Cocaine and amphetamines** — nervousness, hallucinations, tremors, seizures, rapid pulse, high blood pressure, loss of consciousness, dry mouth, dilated pupils.
- **LSD** — confusion, hallucinations, dilated pupils, rapid pulse, loss of consciousness, dry mouth.
- **Narcotics** (codeine, morphine, heroin) — nausea and vomiting, constipation, confusion, sleepiness, loss of consciousness, pinpoint pupils, slow, shallow breathing.
- **Marijuana** — confusion, sedation, nausea and vomiting, loss of consciousness.

WHAT TO DO FOR PREVENTION
If your child is being treated with one of those drugs (e.g., codeine or morphine for cancer), be sure to discuss with your physician and pharmacist the exact dose the child needs, the interactions that may occur with other drugs, and side effects of chronic use. Be extremely careful to give the correct dose when switching from liquid to tablets or capsules, and vice versa.

WHAT TO DO IN CASE OF POISONING

1. Remove remaining tablets from mouth.
2. Ensure that the child is breathing and has a heartbeat (see page 3).
3. Induce vomiting with ipecac (see page 5). If the child is sleepy, unconscious, already vomiting, or has had a seizure, do not give ipecac.
4. Take the child to hospital as soon as possible.
5. Bring with you a sample of the drug and try to estimate how much the child has swallowed.

****STRYCHNINE

USE
Strychnine is a compound used to kill rodents.

LEVEL OF DANGER
Strychnine is a very dangerous material. Even a tiny amount can kill a child. It has no place in your household.

SIGNS OF POISONING (not all signs have to be present)
Stiffening of knees upon walking, spasm (tightness) of muscles, seizures, difficulty in breathing.

WHAT TO DO IN CASE OF POISONING
1. Remove remaining material from mouth.
2. Ensure that the child is breathing and has a heartbeat (see page 3).
3. Induce vomiting with ipecac (see page 5). If the child is sleepy, unconscious, already vomiting, or has had a seizure, do not give ipecac.
4. Take the child to hospital as soon as possible.
5. Bring with you the chemical and try to estimate how much the child has swallowed.

****THEOPHYLLINE

COMMERCIAL NAMES
Accurbon, Aeralate, Aquaphyllin, Azpan, Bronkodyl, Constant-T, Duraphyl, Elixophyllin, Lodrane, Maraz, Mudrane, Primatene, Quibron, Respbid, Slo-Bid, Slo-Phyllin, Somophyllin, Sustaire, Synophylate, Tedral, Theo-24, Theobid, Theochron, Theo-Dur, Theofedral, Theolair, Theo-SR, Theovent, Uniphyl.

USE
Theophylline is used in the treatment of asthma. It is also used to treat apnoea (a temporary inability to breathe) in newborn infants.

LEVEL OF DANGER
Just one adult-strength tablet of theophylline can be fatal to a small child.

SIGNS OF POISONING (not all signs have to be present)
Nausea and vomiting, nervousness, loss of consciousness, convulsions, irregularities of heartbeat.

WHAT TO DO FOR PREVENTION
If your child is being treated with this drug, be sure to discuss with your physician and pharmacist the exact dose the child needs, the interactions that may occur with other drugs, and side effects of chronic use. Be extremely careful to give the correct dose when switching from liquid to tablets or capsules, and vice versa.

WHAT TO DO IN CASE OF POISONING
1. Remove remaining tablets from mouth.
2. Ensure that the child is breathing and has a heartbeat (see page 3).
3. Induce vomiting with ipecac (see page 5). If the child is sleepy, unconscious, already vomiting, or has had a seizure, do not give ipecac.
4. Take the child to hospital as soon as possible.
5. Bring with you the drug container and try to estimate how much the child has swallowed.

**VALPROIC ACID

COMMERCIAL NAMES
Depakene.

USE
Valproic acid is a drug for various types of epilepsy, used by many adults and children.

LEVEL OF DANGER
Valproic acid can be life-threatening to a child. Eight 250-mg tablets are dangerous to a 10-kg (22 lb) toddler.

SIGNS OF POISONING (not all signs have to be present)
Nausea and vomiting, signs of bleeding (e.g., skin). Decrease in level of consciousness (i.e., drowsiness, sleepiness, unresponsiveness), slow, shallow respiration, grey-blue skin due to lack of oxygen (cyanosis), cold skin, liver failure.

WHAT TO DO FOR PREVENTION
If your child is being treated with valproic acid, be sure to discuss with your physician or pharmacist the exact dose the child needs, the interactions that may occur with other drugs, and side effects of chronic use. Be extremely careful to give the correct dose when switching from liquid to tablets, or vice versa.

WHAT TO DO IN CASE OF POISONING
1. Remove remaining tablets from mouth.
2. Ensure that the child is breathing and has a heartbeat (see page 3).
3. Induce vomiting with ipecac (see page 5). If the child is sleepy, unconscious, already vomiting, or has had a seizure, do not give ipecac.
4. Take the child to hospital as soon as possible.
5. Bring with you the drug container and try to estimate how much the child has swallowed.

*VITAMINS

USE

Vitamin tablets are given as supplementary nutrition.

LEVEL OF DANGER

If the brand of vitamin does not contain iron, even a large number of vitamin pills is not likely to be life-threatening to a child. However, if pills contain iron, then ingestion can be very dangerous. (See Iron Preparations, page 71.)

SIGNS OF POISONING (not all signs have to be present)

A one-time ingestion will rarely cause signs of toxicity. Vitamin A can cause headache, and vitamin C, diarrhea.

WHAT TO DO FOR PREVENTION

If your child takes vitamin pills regularly, be sure to discuss with your physician or pharmacist signs of chronic toxicity.

WHAT TO DO IN CASE OF POISONING

If the pill does not contain iron, call your physician or poison control centre, but *do not* induce vomiting.

***YEW

BACKGROUND
The yew is an evergreen tree or shrub. Its bark, wood, leaves, and seeds contain the poison taxine.

LEVEL OF DANGER
Ingestion of several leaves can be life-threatening to a small child.

SIGNS OF POISONING (not all signs have to be present)
Nausea, vomiting, diarrhea, stomach pain, difficulty in breathing, weakness, seizure, loss of consciousness, and dilated pupils.

WHAT TO DO IN CASE OF POISONING
1. Remove remaining plant from mouth.
2. Ensure that the child is breathing and has a heartbeat (see page 3).
3. Induce vomiting with ipecac (see page 5). If the child is sleepy, unconscious, already vomiting, or has had a seizure, do not give ipecac.
4. Take the child to hospital as soon as possible.
5. Bring with you a plant sample and try to estimate how much the child has swallowed.

APPENDIX

POISON CONTROL
CENTERS

UNITED STATES

Akron Regional Poison Center
Childrens' Hospital Medical Center of Akron
281 Locust Street
Akron, OH 44308
Emergency Tel: (216) 379-8562
(800) 362-9922 (OH only)

Alabama Poison Center
809 University Boulevard East
Tuscaloosa, AL 35401
Emergency Tel: (800) 462-0800 (AL only)
(205) 345-0600

Anchorage Poison Control Center
Providence Hospital
3200 Providence Drive
PO Box 196604
Anchorage, Alaska 99519-6604
Emergency Tel: (907) 261-3193
(800) 478-3193

Arizona Poison and Drug Information Center
1501 North Campbell Ave.
Room 3204-K
Tucson, AZ 85724
Emergency Tel: (602) 626-6016
(800) 362-0101 (AZ only)

Arkansas Poison and Drug Information Center
University of Arkansas for Medical Sciences
4301 West Markham Street, Slot 522
Little Rock, AR 72205
Emergency Tel: (501) 666-5532
(800) 482-8948

Bethesda Poison Control Center
Bethesda Hospital
2951 Maple Avenue
Zanesville, OH 43701
Emergency Tel: (614) 454-4221

Bixby Poison Center
Emma L. Bixby Medical Center
818 Riverside Avenue
Adrian, MI 49221
Emergency Tel: (517) 263-2412

Blodgett Regional Poison Center
Blodgett Memorial Medical Center
1840 Wealthy, S.E.
Grand Rapids, MI 49506
Emergency Tel: (800) 632-2727

Blue Ridge Poison Center
Blue Ridge Hospital
University of Virginia
Wright Building, Third Floor
PO Box 67
Charlottesville, VA 22901
Emergency Tel: (800) 451-1428

BroMenn Poison Control Center
Brokaw Hospital (BroMenn Health Care)
Franklin at Virginia
Normal, IL 61761
Emergency Tel: (309) 454-6666

Capital Area Poison Center
University Hospital
The Milton S. Hershey Medical Center
500 University Drive
Hershey, PA 17033
Emergency Tel: (717) 531-6111

Cardinal Glennon Children's Hospital
Regional Poison Control Center
1465 South Grand Boulevard
St. Louis, MO 63104
Emergency Tel: (800) 392-9111
　　　　　　　　(800) 366-8888
　　　　　　　　(314) 772-5200

Catawba Memorial Hospital Poison Control Center
Catawba Memorial Hospital
810 Fairgrove Church Road
Hickory, NC 28602
Emergency Tel: (704) 322-6649

Central New York Poison Control Center
SUNY Health Sciences Center at Syracuse
750 East Adams Street
Syracuse, NY 13210
Emergency Tel: (315) 476-4766
　　　　　　　　(800) 252-5655

Central Ohio Poison Center
Children's Hospital
700 Children's Drive
Columbus, OH 43205
Emergency Tel: (800) 682-7625
　　　　　　　　(614) 228-1323

Central Virginia Poison Center
Medical College of Virginia Hospitals
401 North 12th Street
Richmond, VA 23298-0522
Emergency Tel: (804) 786-9123
　　　　　　　　(call collect)

Central Washington Poison Center
Yakima Valley Memorial Hospital
2811 Tieton Drive
Yakima, WA 98902
Emergency Tel: (509) 248-4400
              (800) 572-9176

Chicago and Northeastern Illinois
Regional Poison Control Center
Rush-Presbyterian-St. Luke's Medical Center
1653 West Congress Parkway
Chicago, IL 60612
Emergency Tel: (312) 942-5969
              (800) 942-5969 (IL only)

Children's Hospital of Alabama Regional Poison Center
The Children's Hospital of Alabama
1600 7th Avenue South
Birmingham, AL 35233-1711
Emergency Tel: (205) 939-9201
              (205) 933-4050
              (800) 292-6678

Children's Hospital of Michigan Poison Control Center
3901 Beaubien Boulevard
Detroit, MI 48201
Emergency Tel: (313) 745-5711
              (800) 462-6642 (MI only)

Children's Mercy Hospital
24th and Gillham Roads
Kansas City, MO 64108
Emergency Tel: (816) 234-3000

Clinical Toxicology Service
University Medical Center
655 West 8th Street
Jacksonville, FL 32209
Emergency Tel: (904) 350-6899

Connecticut Poison Control Center
University of Connecticut Health Center
Farmington Avenue
Farmington, CT 06032
Emergency Tel: (800) 343-2722

Delaware Valley Regional Poison Control Program
34th Street and Civic Center Boulevard
One Children's Center
Philadelphia, PA 19104-4303
Emergency Tel: (215) 386-2100

Duke University Poison Control Center
Duke University Medical Center
PO Box 3007
Durham, NC 27710
Emergency Tel: (919) 684-4438
(800) 672-1697 (NC only)

El Paso Poison Control Center
Thomason Hospital
4815 Alameda Avenue
El Paso, TX 79998
Emergency Tel: (915) 533-1244

Finger Lakes Regional Poison Control Center at Life Line
601 Elmwood Avenue
Rochester, NY 14642
Emergency Tel: (716) 275-5151

**The Florida Poison Information Center
at Tampa General Hospital**
Davis Island
PO Box 1289
Tampa, FL 33601
Emergency Tel: (813) 253-4444
(800) 282-3171 (FL only)

Forrest General Hospital
400 South 28th Avenue
Hattiesburg, MS 39402
Emergency Tel: (601) 288-4235
(601) 288-4236

Fresno Regional Poison Control Center
Fresno Community Hospital and Medical Center
2823 Fresno Street
Fresno, CA 93721
Emergency Tel: (209) 445-1222

The Georgia Poison Control Center
Grady Memorial Hospital
80 Butler Street, SE
Atlanta, GA 30335-3801
Emergency Tel: (404) 589-4400

Greater Cleveland Poison Control Center
University Hospitals of Cleveland
2101 Adelbert Road
Cleveland, OH 44106
Emergency Tel: (216) 231-4455

Green Bay Poison Center
St. Vincent Hospital
835 South Van Buren
Green Bay, WI 54307-3508
Emergency Tel: (414) 433-8100

Hamot Poison Information Center
Hamot Medical Center
201 State Street
Erie, PA 16550
Emergency Tel: (814) 870-6111
Extension 6112

Hawaii Poison Information Center
Kapiolani Medical Center for Women and Children
1319 Punahou Street
Honolulu, Hawaii 96826
Emergency Tel: (808) 941-4411

Hennepin Regional Poison Center
Hennepin County Medical Center
701 Park Avenue South
Minneapolis, MN 55415
Emergency Tel: (612) 347-3141

Hudson Valley Poison Center
Nyack Hospital
160 North Midland Avenue
Nyack, NY 10960
Emergency Tel: (914) 353-1000
              (800) 336-6997

Idaho Poison Control Center
Saint Alphonsus Regional Medical Center
1055 North Curtis Road
Boise, ID 83706
Emergency Tel: (800) 632-8000

Indiana Poison Center
Methodist Hospital of Indiana, Inc.
1701 North Senate Boulevard
Indianapolis, Indiana 46206
Emergency Tel: (800) 382-9097
              (317) 929-2323

Intermountain Regional Poison Control Center
University of Utah
50 North Medical Drive, Building 528
Salt Lake City, UT 84132
Emergency Tel: (800) 456-7707 (UT only)
              (801) 581-2151

Kentucky Regional Poison Center of Kosair Children's Hospital
315 East Broadway
Louisville, KY 40232-5070
Emergency Tel: (502) 589-8222
              (800) 722-5725 (KY only)

Keystone Region Poison Center
Mercy Hospital
2500 7th Avenue
Altoona, PA 16603
Emergency Tel: (814) 946-3711

La Crosse Area Poison Center
St. Francis Medical Center
700 West Avenue South
La Crosse, WI 54601
Emergency Tel: (608) 785-0940

Lehigh Valley Poison Center
The Allentown Hospital
17th and Chew streets
Allentown, PA 18102
Emergency Tel: (215) 433-2311

Long Island Regional Poison Control Center
Nassau County Medical Center
2201 Hempstead Turnpike
East Meadow, NY 11554
Emergency Tel: (516) 542-2323
              (516) 542-2324
              (516) 542-2325
              (516) 542-3813 (TTY)

Los Angeles County Medical Association
Regional Poison Control Center
1925 Wilshire Boulevard
Los Angeles, CA 90057
Emergency Tel: (213) 484-5151
              (213) 664-2121

Mahoning Valley Poison Center
St. Elizabeth Hospital Medical Center
1044 Belmont Avenue
Youngstown, OH 44501
Emergency Tel: (216) 746-2222
(800) 426-2348
(216) 746-5510

Maine Poison Control Center
Maine Medical Center
22 Bramhall Street
Portland, ME 04102
Emergency Tel: (207) 871-2950

Mary Bridge Poison Center
Multicare Medical Center
317 South K Street
Tacoma, WA 98405-0986
Emergency Tel: (206) 594-1414
(800) 542-6319 (WA only)

Maryland Poison Center
University of Maryland School of Pharmacy
20 North Pine Street
Baltimore, MD 21201
Emergency Tel: (301) 528-7701
(800) 492-2414 (MD only)

Massachusetts Poison Control System
The Children's Hospital
300 Longwood Avenue
Boston, MA 02115
Emergency Tel: (617) 232-2120
(800) 682-9211

McKennan Poison Center
McKennan Hospital
800 East 21st Street
Sioux Falls, SD 57117-5045
Emergency Tel: (800) 952-0123 (SD only)
(800) 843-0505
(MN, IA, NE)
(605) 339-7875

Medical Center Hospital Poison Control
Medical Center Hospital
504 Medical Center Boulevard
Conroe, TX 77305
Emergency Tel: (409) 539-7700

Mercy Hospital Poison Control Center
Mercy Hospital Inc.
2001 Vail Avenue
Charlotte, NC 28207
Emergency Tel: (704) 379-5827

**Middle Tennessee Regional Poison
and Clinical Toxicology Center**
Vanderbilt University Medical Center
501 Oxford House
1313 Twenty-First Avenue South
Nashville, TN 37212
Emergency Tel: (615) 322-6435
(800) 288-9999 (TN only)

Mid-America Poison Control Center
Kansas University Medical Center
39th and Rainbow Boulevard
Room B-400 Bell
Kansas City, KS 66103
Emergency Tel: (913) 588-6633
(800) 332-6633 (KS only)

Mid-Plains Poison Center
Children's Memorial Hospital
8301 Dodge Street
Omaha, NE 68114
Emergency Tel: (402) 390-5555
(Omaha only)
(800) 955-9119
(NE and surrounding states)

Milwaukee Poison Center
Children's Hospital of Wisconsin
9000 West Wisconsin
Milwaukee, WI 53201
Emergency Tel: (414) 266-2222

Minnesota Regional Poison Center
St. Paul-Ramsey Medical Center
640 Jackson Street
St. Paul, MN 55101
Emergency Tel: (612) 221-2113

Mississippi Regional Poison Control
University of Mississippi Medical Center
2500 North State Street
Jackson, MS 39216
Emergency Tel: (601) 354-7660

National Capital Poison Center
Georgetown University Hospital
3800 Reservoir Road, NW
Washington, DC 20007
Emergency Tel: (202) 625-3333
(202) 784-4660 (TTY)

New Hampshire Poison Information Center
Dartmouth-Hitchcock Medical Center
2 Maynard Street
Hanover, NH 03756
Emergency Tel: (603) 646-5000

New Jersey Poison Information and Education System
201 Lyons Avenue
Newark, NJ 07112
Emergency Tel: (800) 962-1253

New Mexico Poison and Drug Information Center
The University of New Mexico
2400 Marble Street
Albuquerque, NM 87131
Emergency Tel: (505) 843-2551
(800) 432-6866 (NM only)

New York City Poison Control Center
New York City Department of Health
455 First Avenue, Room 123
New York, NY 10016
Emergency Tel: (212) POISONS
(212) 340-4494

New York State Department of Health
ESP Corning Tower Building, Room 621
Empire State Plaza
Albany, NY 12237
Emergency Tel: (518) 473-1143

North Dakota Poison Information Center
St. Luke's Hospitals-MeritCare
720 4th Street North
Fargo, ND 58122
Emergency Tel: (701) 234-5575
(800) 732-2200 (ND only)

North Texas Poison Center
Parkland Memorial Hospital
5201 Harry Hines Boulevard
Dallas, TX 75235
Emergency Tel: (214) 590-5000
(800) 441-0040 (TX only)

Northwest Regional Poison Center
Saint Vincent Health Center
232 West 25th Street
Erie, PA 16544
Emergency Tel: (814) 452-3232
(800) 822-3232

Oklahoma Poison Control Center
Oklahoma Medical Center
940 NE 13th
Oklahoma City, OH 73126
Emergency Tel: (405) 271-5454
(800) 522-4611 (OK only)

Oregon Poison Center
Oregon Health Sciences University
3181 SW Sam Jackson Park Road, UHN 2521
Portland, OR 97201
Emergency Tel: (503) 279-8968
(800) 452-7165 (OR only)

Palmetto Poison Center
University of South Carolina
Sumter Street
Columbia, SC 29208
Emergency Tel: (803) 765-7359
(800) 922-1117 (SC only)

Pittsburgh Poison Center
Children's Hospital of Pittsburgh
3705 Fifth Avenue at DeSoto St.
Pittsburgh, PA 15213
Emergency Tel: (412) 681-6669

**Regional Poison Control System and
Cincinnati Drug and Poison Information Center**
University of Cincinnati Medical Center
231 Bethesda Avenue, M.L. 144
Cincinnati, OH 45267-0144
Emergency Tel: (513) 558-5111

Regional Poison Resource Center
Pekin Memorial Hospital
Court and 14th Streets
Pekin, IL 61554
Emergency Tel: (309) 353-0430

Rocky Mountain Poison and Drug Center
Department of Health and Hospital
645 Bannock Street
Denver, CO 80204-4507
Emergency Tel: (303) 629-1123
        (800) 332-3073 (CO only)
        (880) 442-2702 (WY only)
        (800) 525-9083 (MT only)

Rhode Island Poison Center
Rhode Island Hospital
593 Eddy Street
Providence, RI 02903
Emergency Tel: (401) 277-5727

Saginaw Region Poison Center
Saginaw General Hospital
1447 North Harrison Street
Saginaw, MI 48602
Emergency Tel: (517) 755-1111
        (800) 451-4585

Samaritan Regional Poison Center
Good Samaritan Medical Center
1130 East McDowell Road, Suite A-5
Phoenix, AZ 85006
Emergency Tel: (602) 253-3334

San Diego Regional Poison Center
UCSD Medical Center
225 Dickinson Street, H-925
San Diego, CA 92103-1990
Emergency Tel: (619) 543-6000
        (800) 876-4766

San Francisco Bay Area Regional Poison Control Center
San Francisco General Hospital Medical Center
1001 Potrero Avenue, Room 1-E-86
San Francisco, CA 94110
Emergency Tel: (415) 476-6600
(800) 523-2222 (CA only)

Santa Clara Valley Medical Center Regional Poison Center
751 South Bascom Avenue
San Jose, CA 95128
Emergency Tel: (408) 299-5112
(800) 662-9886

Savannah Regional/EMS Poison Control Center
Memorial Medical Center, Inc.
4700 Waters Avenue
Savannah, GA 31403
Emergency Tel: (912) 355-5228

Seattle Poison Center
Children's Hospital and Medical Center
4800 Sand Point Way, NE
Seattle, WA 98105
Emergency Tel: (206) 526-2121
(880) 732-6985 (WA only)

Southern Poison Center, Inc.
848 Adams Avenue
Memphis, TN 38103
Emergency Tel: (901) 528-6048

Southwest Virginia Poison Center
Roanoke Memorial Hospitals
Belleview at Jefferson Street
Roanoke, VA 24033
Emergency Tel: (703) 981-7336

Spokane Poison Center
Empire Health Consolidated Services
715 South Cowley
Spokane, WA 99202
Emergency Tel: (509) 747-1077

Stark County Poison Control Center
Timken Mercy Medical Center
1320 Timken Mercy Drive, NW
Canton, OH 44708
Emergency Tel: (800) 722-8662

**St. John's Hospital Regional Poison Resource Center
for Central and Southern Illinois**
St. John's Hospital
800 East Carpenter
Springfield, IL 62769
Emergency Tel: (217) 753-3330
             (800) 252-2022

St. Joseph Hospital and Health Care Center
250 College Avenue
Lancaster, PA 17604
Emergency Tel: (717) 291-8111

St. Luke's Midland Regional Medical Center
305 South State Street
Aberdeen, SD 57401
Emergency Tel: (605) 622-5100

St. Luke's Poison Center
St. Luke's Regional Medical Center
2720 Stone Park Boulevard
Sioux City, IA 51104
Emergency Tel: (712) 277-2222
             (800) 352-2222

St. Vincent's Medical Center Poison Control Center
1800 Barrs Street
Jacksonville, FL 32203
Emergency Tel: (904) 387-7500

Susquehanna Poison Center
Geisinger Medical Center
North Academy Avenue
Danville, PA 17821
Emergency Tel: (717) 271-6116
              (717) 275-6116

Terrebonne General Medical Center
Drug and Poison Information Service
936 East Main Street
Hourma, LA 70360
Emergency Tel: (504) 873-4067
              (504) 873-4066

Texas State Poison Center
The University of Texas Medical Branch
Clinical Science Building, Room 1202
Galveston, TX 77550-2780
Emergency Tel: (409) 765-1420
              (713) 654-1701
              (800) 392-8548 (TX only)

Triad Poison Center
The Moses H. Cone Memorial Hospital
1200 North Elm Street
Greensboro, NC 27401-1020
Emergency Tel: (919) 379-4105
              (800) 722-2222 (NC only)

University of California
Davis Medical Center
Regional Poison Control Center
2315 Stockton Boulevard, Room 1151
Sacramento, CA 95817
Emergency Tel: (916) 734-3692
(800) 342-9293

University Hospital Poison Control Center
4301 W. Markham, Mail Slot 584
Little Rock, AR 72205-7199
Emergency Tel: (501) 661-6161

University of Wisconsin Regional Poison Center
600 Highland Avenue, E5/238 CSC
Madison, WI 53792
Emergency Tel: (608) 262-3702

UC Irvine Regional Poison Center
University of California Irvine Medical Center
101 The City Drive, Route 78
Orange, CA 92668
Emergency Tel: (714) 634-5988
(800) 544-4404
(Southern CA only)

Variety Club Poison and Drug Information Center
Iowa Methodist Medical Center
1200 Pleasant Street
Des Moines, IA 50309
Emergency Tel: (800) 362-2327

Vermont Poison Center
Medical Center Hospital of Vermont
111 Colchester Avenue
Burlington, VT 05401
Emergency Tel: (802) 658-3456

West Virginia Poison Center
West Virginia University School of Pharmacy
3110 MacCorkle Avenue, SE
Charleston, WV 25304
Emergency Tel: (304) 348-4211 (local)
            (800) 642-3625 (WV only)

Western New York Regional Poison Control Center
Children's Hospital of Buffalo
219 Bryant Street
Buffalo, NY 14226
Emergency Tel: (716) 878-7654

Western Ohio Poison and Drug Information Center
Children's Medical Center
One Children's Plaza
Dayton, OH 45404-1815
Emergency Tel: (513) 222-2227
            (800) 762-0727 (OH only)

W.A. Foote Memorial Hospital
205 North East Avenue
Jackson, MI 49201
Business Tel: (517) 788-4816
Emergency Tel: (517) 788-4811

INDEX

Antislene, 31
Antituberculosis drugs, 73
Antrocal, 92
Apnoea, 108
Apo-Carbamazepine, 40
Apo-Primidone, 26
Aposazide, 33
Apoval, 56
Apples, 49
Apresoline, 33
Apricots, 49
Aquaphyllin, 108
Aquatensen, 54
Aralen, 35
Arco-Lase, 29
Arsenic, 57
Arthrinal, 37
Artificial respiration, 3
Arum, 36
ASA, 37
Asasantine, 37
Ascofer, 71
Ascriptin, 37
Asendin, 19
Aspirin, 37, 11, 47, 86
Asthma, 108
Astin, 37
Atrax, 31
Atrohist, 31
Auentyl, 87
Automobile, 13
Azpan, 92
Azpan, 108

BAC, 99
Bacid, 29
Bacillus cereus, 61
Bacteria, 22, 61, 101
Bactrim, 22
Bancap, 11, 84
Banex, 11
Bantrol, 43
Banvel, 43
Barium sulfide, 46
Barnon, 43
Bath oil, 9
Batteries, 16, 39, 74
Battery burning, 74

Battery fluid, 13
Bed wetting, 70
Belianderal, 92
Bellanderal, 92
Beminal Stress, 71
Benadryl, 31, 47, 99
Benylin, 47
Benzene hexachloride, 43
Benzene, 14, 57, 91
Betaloc, 33
Bidigin, 43
Bienoxane, 24
Biquin, 20
Blazer, 43
Bleach, 2
Bleaches, 13, 16
Blighia sophida, 15
Blocraden, 33
Blood thinner, 37
Body lotion, 9
Botulism, 61
Bravo, 43
Breathing, 3
Breoprin, 37
Bretylol, 20
Bromfed, 31, 47
Bromophos, 88
Bronkodyl, 108
Brown recluse spider, 104
Bufferin, 37
Bullet retention, 74
Bumex, 54
Butacarb, 88

Cabinets, 1
Caladium, 36
Calamine lotion, 9
Calan, 20, 33
Calcidrine, 47
Calfrate, 71
Calla lily, 36
Calocasia, 36
Cals Cogeopinin, 11
Camcolit, 75
Cancer, 80, 82
Candles, 9
Capoten, 33
Capozide, 33, 54

134

Cough, 47
CPR, 2
Crayons, 9
Creams, 10
Crystodigin, 51
Curatin, 56
Cuticle remover, 46
Cyanide, 49
Cyanophos, 88
Cytosar, 24
Cytoxan, 24

Dalmane, 99
Dama. Blanca, 105
Damcet, 11
Darvocet, 11, 96
Darvon, 96
DDT, 43
Declinax, 33
Deconamine, 31, 47
Deconil, 43
Decontamination, 5
Delensol, 20
Demolox, 19
Demosan, 43
Deodorants, 10
Deodorizers, 10
Depakene, 26, 109
Depilatories, 46
Depression, 40, 87
Depressive disorders, 18, 19, 28, 50,
    56, 70, 77
Deralin, 20
Dermoplast, 76
Desipramine, 28, 50
Desyrel, 28
Diabenese, 69
DiaBeta, 69
Diabetes mellitus, 69
Dialysis, 7
Diamox, 54
Diarrhea, 7, 29
Diazinon, 88
Diban, 29
Diesel oil, 91
Digitalis, 51
Digitalis-producing plants, 52
Digoxin, 51, 52

Dilantin, 26, 93
Dilaudid, 47, 84
Dimedrine, 47
Dimetan, 88
Dimetane, 31, 45
Dimetapp, 31, 47
Dimilin, 43
Dionin, 84
Dioxin, 53
Diphenoxylate, 84
Diphenylhydantoin, 93
Dirrelor, 69
Dishwasher detergents, 16
Diucardin, 54
Diulo, 54
Diupres, 33
Diuretics, 54
Diuril, 54
Diurtensen, 54
Diutensen, 33
Dog parsley, 67
Dolecet, 11
Dolobid, 86
Dolophine, 84
Dolophine Hydrochloride,
    80
Dolprin, 37, 45
Domical, 18
Donnagel-MB, 29
Dope, 105
Dorcol, 11, 47
Doxepin, 28, 56
Doxycycline, 22
Drain cleaners, 2, 13, 16
Dristan, 11, 31, 37, 47
Drixoral, 31
Drixoral, 47
Drixtab, 47
Drugs, 1, 17
Dura-tabs, 20
Duralith, 75
Duraphyl, 108
Duraquin, 20
Dureticyl, 54
Durrax, 31
Dyazide, 33
Dyazide, 54
Dyes, 57

Largon, 99
Lasix, 54
Laxatives, 10
Lead, 74
Leaden pots, 74
Lentanyl, 105
Leritine, 84
Levate, 18
Levazine, 18
Librium, 99
Lidocaine, 20, 76
Lighter fluids, 6
Lily of the valley, 52
Limas, 75
Lindane, 43
Lipstick, 10
Liquid detergent, 6
Liquid lady, 105
Lithane, 75
Lithium, 75
Lithizine, 75
Lithobid, 75
Lithonate, 75
Local anaesthetics, 76
Lodrane, 108
Lomotil, 29, 84
Loniten, 33
Lopressor, 33
Lortab, 11
Lortab ASA, 37
Lotion, 10
Lozol, 54
Lubraseptic, 76
Lubricants, 10
Lubricating oils, 91
Ludiomil, 77
Lumbitrol, 18
Luminal, 92
Lungs, 5, 8
Lupus erythematosus, 24, 35
Lye, 2

Maintain, 43
Make-up, 10
Malaria, 35
Malathion, 88
Malema, 71
Maltlevol, 71

Manic-depressive disorders, 75
Maprotiline, 77
Maprotiline, 28
Maraz, 108
Mataven, 43
Matches, 10
Maxzide, 54
Medilgeric, 11
Mediphen, 92
Medomen, 86
Melipamin, 70
Meningitis, 97
Mepergan, 99
Mercuric oxide, 39
Mercury, 78
Metal cleaners, 13, 16
Metal cleaning, 49
Metallic mercury, 78
Metals, 79
Metatensin, 33
Methadone, 80
Methadone Hydrochloride, 80
Methane, 81
Methotrexate, 24
Mevanin, 71
Mexate, 24
Mexitil, 20
Micronase, 69
Midamor, 54
Midol, 11, 37
Migraines, 86
Migralam, 11
Mineral oil, 10
Mineral spirit, 91
Minipress, 33
Minizide, 33
Mithracin, 24
Mitrolan, 29
Mobenol, 69
Moduret, 33, 54
Moduretic, 54
Mogadone, 99
Morning sickness, 31
Morphine, 82
Motrin, 86
Mouth, 6
Mouth-to-mouth resuscitation, 3
Mouth-to-mouth respiration, 4